D0853480

POISONS ON OUR PLATES

POISONS
— ON OUR PLATES —

The Real Food Safety Problem
in the United States

MICHELE MORRONE

Politics and the Environment
P. H. Liotta, Series Editor

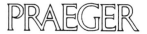

Westport, Connecticut
London

RWC
RA
1258
.M66
2008

Library of Congress Cataloging-in-Publication Data

Morrone, Michele, 1962-
    Poisons on our plates : the real food safety problem in the United States / Michele Morrone.
       p. ; cm. — (Politics and the environment, ISSN 1932-3484)
   Includes bibliographical references and index.
   ISBN 978-0-313-34975-1 (alk. paper)
   1. Food—Toxicology—United States.   2. Food contamination—United States.
3. Food—Microbiology—United States.   4. Food industry and trade—Health aspects—United
States.   I. Title. II. Series.
   [DNLM: 1. Food Contamination—United States.   2. Food Industry—standards—United
States.   3. Food Microbiology—United States. WA 701 M883p 2008]
    RA1258.M66 2008
    363.19'26—dc22   2008010985

British Library Cataloguing in Publication Data is available.

Copyright © 2008 by Michele Morrone

All rights reserved. No portion of this book may be
reproduced, by any process or technique, without the
express written consent of the publisher.

Library of Congress Catalog Card Number: 2008010985

ISBN: 978–0–313–34975–1
ISSN: 1932–3484

First published in 2008

Praeger Publishers, 88 Post Road West, Westport, CT 06881
An imprint of Greenwood Publishing Group, Inc.
www.praeger.com

Printed in the United States of America

The paper used in this book complies with the
Permanent Paper Standard issued by the National
Information Standards Organization (Z39.48–1984).

10 9 8 7 6 5 4 3 2 1

For my family and their healthy appetites

5-15-09 7L 9780313349751

Contents

Series Foreword

The key focus of the Praeger Politics and the Environment series is to explore the interstices between environment, political, and security impacts in the twenty-first century. To those intimately involved with these issues, their immediacy and importance are obvious. What is not obvious to many, nonetheless—including those involved in making decisions that affect our collective future—is how these three critical issues are in constant conflict and frequently clash. Today, more so than at any other time in human history, intersecting environmental, political, and security issues profoundly impact our lives and the lives of those to come.

In examining the complex interdependence of these three impact effects, the study of environmental and security issues should recognize several distinct and pragmatic truths. One, international organizations today are established for and focus best on security issues. Thus, while it remains difficult to address environmental threats, challenges, and vulnerabilities for these organizations, it makes eminently better sense to reform what we have rather than constantly invent the "new" organization that may be no better equipped to handle current and future challenges. Secondly, new protocols must continue to be created, worked into signature, and managed under the leadership of states through international organizations and cooperative regimes. Finally, and incorporating the reality of these previous two truths, we should honestly recognize that environmental challenges can best be presented in terms that relate to security issues. To that end, it is sensible to depict environmental challenges in language that is understandable to decision makers most familiar with security impacts and issues.

There is benefit and danger in this approach, of course. Not all security issues involve direct threats; some security issues, as with some political processes, are far more nuanced, more subtle, and less clearly evident. I would argue further—as I have been arguing for several decades now—that it remains a tragic mistake to couch all security issues in terms of threat. To the contrary, what I term "creeping vulnerabilities"—climate change; population growth; disease; scarcity of water and other natural resources; decline in food production, access, and availability; soil erosion and desertification; urbanization and pollution; and the lack of effective warning systems—can come to have a far more devastating impact effect if such issues are ignored and left unchecked over time. In the worst possible outcomes, vulnerabilities left unchecked over time *will* manifest themselves as threats.

In its most direct, effective, and encompassing assessment, environmental security centers on a focus that seeks the best response to changing environmental conditions that have the potential to reduce stability and affect peaceful relationships, and—if left unchecked—could lead to the outbreak of conflict. This working definition, therefore, represents the vital core of the Praeger Politics and the Environment series.

This latest volume of the Politics and the Environment series, nonetheless, offers the most human—and, in many ways, the most terrifying—impact that careless environmental conditions create and the "blowback" that consumers experience when neglect and inattention occur. In a word, Michele Morrone's *Poisons on Our Plates* is shocking.

Morrone's work is meticulously researched and immensely readable, and will broaden and deepen the Politics and the Environment Series significantly. Although one could easily be sent reeling from the grotesque horrors that Morrone describes with precision, there is a light touch as well to the work that makes for a compelling, powerful narrative. Indeed, just as the book *Fast Food Nation* and the film *Super Size Me* had a profound impact on the way people viewed the convenience as well as the dangers of fast food, Morrone points to the abuse and the risks that surround what we commonly believe are safe nutritional practices. Indeed, as she underscores throughout the work, the dangers of pandemic influenza, bacteria, and viruses are far more threatening and direct than the risks of terrorism or nuclear war.

Environmentalists often predict that an apocalypse is coming: The earth will heat up like a greenhouse. We will run out of energy. Overpopulation will lead to starvation and war. Nuclear winter will devastate all organic life. We have, of course, grown desensitized to many such prophecies of doom. Yet as this work suggests with brilliant clarity, the real danger is already here—at dinnertime.

P. H. Liotta
Executive Director
Pell Center for International Relations and Public Policy
Salve Regina University
Newport, Rhode Island

Introduction

What are you afraid of? Terrorism? Cancer? Flying in an airplane? How about bacteria? If you are like most Americans, you probably are more afraid of dying from cancer than dying from diarrhea. There are real reasons that this is the case, including the fact that cancer is more exotic than diarrhea and less familiar to us; most of us perceive diarrhea as curable and cancer as incurable. Cancer is a chronic condition and diarrhea is something that you can generally get over in a short period of time. The differences in the nature of these two illnesses affect our perception of the risk they represent to us.

We have data that show that the risk of dying from diarrhea in the United States is just not that high—that is, compared with other countries. In the United States, as in other developed countries, we have access to clean drinking water and safe food, and antidiarrheal medications. But if we widen our perspective to an international view, we learn that diarrhea causes more than 2 million deaths worldwide and most of those who die are children. About half of those deaths can be attributed to contaminated water and the other half to food. All of the cases are associated with organisms that we cannot see with the naked eye, but that are circulating in the environment and evolving to become serious global threats to public health and human security.

This book is about diarrhea, and about vomiting, nausea, headaches, and arthritis. Essentially it is about how human health is affected by eating foods containing organisms that are out of sight, and thus usually out of mind, but that are everywhere in our environment. These ubiquitous organisms are microbiological creatures and they include bacteria, viruses, parasites, and prions. They are not exotic, or unusual, but they are fascinating. What I found while researching this book is that all of the microorganisms that are the leading causes of foodborne illness have their own compelling stories. These stories include drama in the laboratories where they were discovered, controversy over naming newly discovered organisms, links to major historical events, and public anxiety created when there is a widespread disease outbreak.

Another part of the story tells what we are doing to control microbiological organisms that may contaminate our food. We know that these invisible contaminants cause most foodborne illnesses worldwide. The main problem in the United States is that our food safety system is not well equipped to address these causes and, until recently, the American public did not seem to care. Recent outbreaks involving microbiologicals have sickened thousands of people, killed too many, and caught the attention of the public. Most of these large-scale outbreaks also emphasize the lack of preparedness, the lack of resources, and, in some cases, the outright neglect of our government with respect to protecting Americans from exposure to serious, preventable illness.

The first chapter of this book is a discussion of basic microbiology and its relationship to food safety. I am not a microbiologist, so this is not an extremely detailed account of the science, but its purpose is to enhance your understanding of the nature of microbes. In addition, strategies for controlling microbiological organisms are discussed in this chapter. For example, the remarkable thing about bacteria is that, while they cause so much illness, they are also relatively easy to kill in foods through simple controls such as using a thermometer to ensure that your food is cooked to a high enough temperature. The purpose of presenting some fundamental information about microbiology is to set the stage for the following chapters, which will focus on specific organisms.

Most nutritionists agree that it is important to eat plenty of fresh fruits and vegetables. However, recent outbreaks involving spinach (at least 205 illnesses, three deaths), green onions (more than 600 ill, at least three deaths), and Roma tomatoes (more than 560 illnesses) suggest that sometimes vegetables can do more harm than good. In chapter 2, I note that fresh produce is not something that we have usually associated with organisms that contaminate hamburgers, but this is changing. Raw sprouts and spinach are two healthy foods that demonstrate the ability of a pathogen usually related to rare hamburger to also contaminate a salad.

Estimates indicate that *Salmonella* bacteria cause about 1.4 million ill-nesses in the United States every year. Four hundred of these people die, which is why I have devoted chapter 3 to this particular pathogen. Some of the more well-known outbreaks of foodborne illness are related to *Salmo-nella* including one of the most notorious outbreaks connected to ice cream consumption in the mid-1990s. It wasn't the ice cream, but egg product that was transported in the truck prior to the ice cream that made more than 2,000 Americans ill. We have usually thought of *Salmonella* as the bug that gets into eggs and chicken, but a recent nationwide outbreak made more than 620 people sick from eating peanut butter. *Salmonella* also has one of the more interesting histories because its background includes questionable scientific integrity and one of the most notorious figures in the history of infectious disease: Typhoid Mary.

I have never been on a cruise, but people tell me that they are quite fun and that it is really easy to gain weight because of the constant availability of food. The other item that is becoming constantly more available on cruises is a virus that could require passengers to spend their voyage in the bath-room rather than the spa. Chapter 4 lays out the history of the Norwalk virus, which is now the leading cause of acute gastrointestinal illness in the United States. Viruses create different challenges than bacteria because of their ability to contaminate virtually anything, including food. The Nor-walk virus was first identified in a small town in Ohio and has become the cause of major outbreaks on cruise ships. As with most viruses, the problem is triggered by poor personal hygiene, and exposures result from food ser-vice workers who do not wash their hands. If ocean waves do not make you queasy on a cruise ship, this chapter might.

In 1993 more than 400,000 people in Milwaukee, Wisconsin had diarrhea at the same time. Their illness was caused by a parasite in drinking water that was treated with chlorine that is supposed to kill infectious agents. Chapter 5 outlines the relationship of clean water to safe food and specifically talks about seafood and salsa, two other healthy foods that have been contami-nated through dirty water. Outbreaks of diseases from dirty water have been linked to public and private water supplies, as well as bottled water. In one recent year, 30 waterborne outbreaks were reported to the Centers for Dis-ease Control and Prevention (CDC) and more than 2,700 Americans were sickened by the microbiologicals in their drinking water.

It is possible to get sick from eating white rice at a Chinese buffet, drinking iced tea served with contaminated ice cubes, or having a turkey sandwich for lunch. Disease outbreaks linked to foods that are considered "ready to eat," such as sandwich meats, suggest that personal hygiene is an important element in ensuring food safety. As chapter 6 explains, there are some serious concerns with foods that we pick up and eat without cooking further. Some of the pathogens that get into these foods cause serious health outcomes, making hot dogs more than just a choking hazard to young children.

Public policy to address microbial food safety in the United States is complicated and uncoordinated. Chapter 7 only scratches the surface of our food safety system by examining several agencies, at all levels of government, that share responsibility. Even with the elaborate and convoluted governmental approach to food safety, ultimately consumers are most responsible for ensuring their own safety. This chapter attempts to explain the more prominent features of the U.S. food safety system and points out its deficiencies in protecting consumers, including a lack of resources and personnel.

When all is said and done, public perception of environmental health risks is the major factor in targeting food safety efforts. Chapter 8 lays out the role that perception played in the cases of Alar on apples and of mad cow disease. Both of these situations are examples of how governmental resources may be targeted toward those issues that may actually pose minimal risk relative to bacteria, viruses, and parasites. In order to improve our food safety system, we need new approaches that target microbial pathogens. Some of these rely on technology, while others are simply political. It is also clear that those responsible for protecting public health from unsafe food need to address the episodic attention that is paid to this issue by lawmakers.

The people who shoulder a major amount of the responsibility for food safety are the local environmental health personnel who inspect restaurants and investigate outbreaks of illness. Throughout the book, there are stories from some of these professionals about outbreak investigations they have been involved in. A few of the stories are rather humorous; others may turn your stomach; but they are all good examples of how easy it is to get sick from eating food that contains the microscopic terrorists known as bacteria, viruses, and parasites.

While researching this book, I became captivated by the scientists who have been pioneers in microbiology. Most of these men were interesting on so many levels, including one who was on an Antarctic expedition, one who was an outspoken critic of Nazism, and one who was dedicated to helping children. All of these scientific pioneers were dedicated to understanding the way in which the smallest organisms on the planet make the biggest impact on human health.

— 1 —

Food Microbiology 101

Who hasn't been disgusted by finding a hair or some other foreign object in their food while eating in a restaurant? Many years ago, while working in a university-area restaurant, I served a tossed salad with a cigarette butt in it. As would be expected, the customer was quite alarmed when she took it out of her mouth. While she stood in the dining room screaming that she was going to get AIDS, it occurred to me that her fears were at least partially accurate because it is not possible to see the organisms that are the most important factors contributing to foodborne illness. We now know that the risk of acquiring AIDS from food is nonexistent, but bacteria, viruses, and parasites in food and water cause millions of illnesses and thousands of deaths every year. Despite our efforts to control these microorganisms, there is evidence that they are evolving to resist some of the tools that have been most effective in killing them in the past.

Evolving microorganisms that are resistant to antibiotics and antivirals are one component of the "perfect storm" that creates major outbreaks of foodborne illness. Other components of this perfect storm include the large scale of food production, increased reliance on imports for fresh food, and the public perception of risk. All three of these components exist under the umbrella of a weakening environmental and public health system. With respect to the scale of food production, one of the best recent examples of how the mass production of food affects our safety can be found in the spinach-related *E. coli* outbreak of 2006. Because of health concerns and the convenience of bagged salads, consumer demand for fresh spinach has increased tremendously in the last 30 years. The U.S. spinach industry reportedly has become a $325 million a year endeavor.[1]

In order to meet the increased demand, fresh spinach is grown at numerous farms and shipped to central processing facilities, where it is all mixed together before it is bagged. This is a common practice in food processing and creates serious challenges to environmental public health professionals when they are involved in an outbreak investigation. One of the primary means of preventing the spread of illness is to quickly identify the cause and trace the suspicious food back to the source. When one bag of spinach contains greens from four or five farms, all of the farms must be investigated. This creates an almost impossible scenario for an environmental public health system that is already stretched beyond its capacity.

The demand for fresh produce year-round has led to the second component of the food danger perfect storm, an increased reliance on imported goods. If you spend a few minutes at your local grocery store looking at your produce, you will find an international smorgasbord of fruits and vegetables. Grapes from Chile, garlic from China, mushrooms from Canada, and apples from New Zealand are just some of the foods we import to keep up with demand. Other imported foods include fresh and frozen fish from China and Vietnam, beef from Canada, and cheeses from all over the world. Even if the food is not contaminated with bacteria or viruses in the country of origin, a lot can happen to a package of flounder on its trip from China to the United States.

The final component of the perfect storm is the lack of public awareness of the impact that microbiological organisms have on the food supply. To compound the problem of the lack of awareness, the public's attention is focused on other dubious threats to the food supply, such as mad cow disease, irradiated food, and genetically modified organisms. History has taught us that public perception is the critical element in the creation of environmental health policy. In the realm of food safety this has translated into inadequate resources to prevent the mundane foodborne illnesses caused by germs, even though these are the greatest imminent threat to our health.

The umbrella that has protected us from the storm, the environmental and public health system in the United States, has some serious holes in it. These holes come in the form of resources diverted away from protecting the public's health from common causes of foodborne illness and to other threats such as bioterrorism and pandemic influenza. While resources are being diverted, the nation's universities are struggling to graduate enough qualified individuals to fill the gaps in an aging public health workforce. Perhaps the one factor that is threatening to turn the umbrella completely inside out is the role that politics play in public health protection.

A BRIEF HISTORY OF THE LEADING CONTENDERS

In order to fully understand the most common causes of foodborne illness and death, it is necessary to have an understanding of basic microbiology. In its simplest form, microbiology is the study of microorganisms such as bacteria and viruses. Microbiology is the basis for some of the more complex sciences, such as molecular biology and biotechnology. It is also the critical foundation for science education because it provides a way in which to examine the interaction among organisms and their environment, also known as the science of ecology.

Hans Schlegel, who was the editor of the *Archives of Microbiology* for 24 years and who is described as a "gifted teacher" who also "made a great impact on non-medical microbiology,"[2] explains the importance of microbiology to science in this way: "Thus, we can compare science progress to walking over a mountainous landscape. Each small discovery is like reaching a new mountaintop, from which we see further peaks that guide our journey.... The best view of biology is that from the peak of general microbiology."[3]

Anyone interested in a history of microbiology should take a look at the book *A Chronology of Microbiology in Historical Context*, by Raymond W. Beck.[4] Beck notes that the first hint that microorganisms might cause illness dates back to 3180 B.C., when there is some evidence of an epidemic tied to an unseen organism. Although his historical account covers hundreds of important events in microbiology, some of the more notable historical events related to food safety include:

- 1070: The discovery that Roquefort cheese was created by a mold
- 1735: First case of foodborne illness recorded
- 1800: Drinking water sanitation begins
- 1804: Canning is used as a way to preserve food
- 1820: A documented outbreak of botulism involving 230 cases
- 1886: Pasteurization of milk begins
- 1894: Several illnesses and one death associated with eating beef contaminated with the *Staphylococci* (staph) bacteria
- 1895: Bacteria identified as the cause of botulism and as the cause of food spoilage in canned foods
- 1896: *Salmonella* confirmed as the cause of death from eating sausage
- 1906: *The Jungle* is published by Upton Sinclair

- 1920–21: Prion disease is discovered by Creutzfeldt and Jakob and named Creutzfeldt-Jakob disease (CJD), now thought to be related to mad cow disease
- 1963: *Campylobacter*, one of the leading causes of foodborne illness, is discovered
- 1982: First outbreaks of foodborne illness associated with *E. coli* O157:H7
- 1990: Cholera epidemic begins in Peru, associated with contaminated shellfish
- 1993: Outbreak of cryptosporidiosis in Milwaukee, Wisconsin associated with contaminated public drinking water

Among the events that are not included in Beck's historical account, but probably will be if a new edition is published, are the outbreaks of Norwalk virus on cruise ships that occurred from 2004 through 2007 and the largest beef recall in U.S. history in spring 2008. As a matter of fact, there may need to be a whole new chapter devoted solely to the year 2007 because of the pet food recall, the outbreak of *E. coli* associated with spinach, the outbreak of salmonellosis associated with peanut butter, and the proposal from the U.S. Congress for a unified food safety agency.

These events are only a few in microbiological history that were milestones in food production and understanding foodborne illness. Throughout this history there were many microbiologists who dedicated their lives to understanding how bacteria, viruses, and parasites get into food and then are transmitted to people. It is interesting that even before there was concrete evidence that microscopic organisms existed in food and were making people sick, processes such as canning were being used to preserve food. Unfortunately, when done incorrectly, canning can cause the most severe type of foodborne illness via a bacterial pathogen that causes botulism.

When a microorganism is capable of causing illness, we refer to it as a "pathogen." Although there is some evidence related to bacteria and viruses as far back as 3000 B.C., the first time that the possibility of microorganisms causing disease was recognized and documented was in 1546, when Girolamo Fracastoro wrote "On Contagion and Contagious Diseases." This work is believed to be the first theoretical discussion about the role that organisms outside of the body play in causing disease. In his writings, Fracastoro set the stage for the science of epidemiology, as he argued that some organisms could be transmitted between people.[5]

Fracastoro's theories were not embraced by other scientists of his time. He followed his book about contagion with one about syphilis, and he is credited with giving this disease its name. His writings about syphilis expounded on how disease can spread from person to person and that some unseen organism was involved in the transmission. It took hundreds of years, but once scientists believed that organisms that could not be seen with the naked eye were capable of making people sick, they began to research ways in which humans were exposed to the organisms.

In 1876, Robert Koch was the first scientist to grow bacteria outside of the human body, a technique known as "culturing." Koch worked with the anthrax bacterium, a pathogen that is transmitted through the air, but his culturing techniques are the foundation for our understanding of the causes of foodborne outbreaks. Koch developed four criteria, or postulates, that are the basis for proving that a specific type of bacteria is the cause of a specific disease:

1. The bacteria must be present in every victim of the disease.
2. The bacteria must be taken from the host with the disease and grown in pure culture.
3. The specific disease must be reproduced when a pure culture of the bacteria is inoculated into a healthy susceptible host.
4. The bacteria must be recoverable from the experimentally infected host.

His postulates lay out the scientific method microbiologists use when attempting to identify the microbiological reasons why people are sick. Adhering to these postulates are critical as environmental health professionals try to pinpoint the causes of foodborne illness. In order to apply them, samples from both the food and victim must be obtained and cultured in a laboratory. Obtaining these samples is one of the more challenging aspects of outbreak investigation. Suspected food has often been discarded well before people are sick, and asking an ill patient for a stool sample is delicate to say the least.

Culturing involves placing very small amounts of a sample on a gel-like substance called "agar" inside of a petri dish. If the bacteria grows into groups, or colonizes, and can be identified as specific bacteria, then Koch's second criterion is fulfilled. By examining the colonies under a microscope, microbiologists can usually classify the organism by its shape.

To further apply Koch's criteria, the colonized bacteria should be inoculated into a healthy host, usually a lab rodent, and then recovered from the host once it becomes ill. Waiting for a healthy host to get sick can take a few hours or up to a month or more depending on the incubation period for the organism to cause disease. Because time is often critical in a foodborne outbreak situation, just being able to grow bacteria in a petri dish from several different samples is usually enough evidence for environmental health officials to declare that the bacteria are the cause of the illness. This allows for a precautionary approach to control the spread of illness to other victims because once the pathogen is identified, appropriate measures can be taken to deal with it.

The late nineteenth and early twentieth centuries were times of great progress in microbiology. New organisms were constantly being discovered and our understanding of how these organisms cause human disease was greatly enhanced. In addition, new techniques for controlling the spread of these germs, such as pasteurization and canning, were implemented. One characteristic of microbiology that makes it so fascinating is that new discoveries are constantly being made. In this way microbiologists are explorers always searching for new and unusual organisms, and this search continues to uncover new organisms today.

Since 1970, microbiologists have identified at least 15 new bacterial pathogens as causes of foodborne illness, including *E. coli* O157:H7 and several new strains of the *Salmonella, Campylobacter,* and *Vibrio* bacteria.[6] There are several reasons why we are discovering new pathogens more rapidly than ever before. These reasons include advances in our technical, research, and surveillance capacities. However, we must consider other factors that may not be related to scientific research and are more policy-oriented. These include factors such as our overreliance on and misuse of antibiotics, farming methods that create conditions conducive to the spread of microbiological organisms, international trade, and public awareness. It is clear that solving our major food safety problem, controlling microbiological pathogens, is complex, involving both scientific and policy approaches.

Microorganisms are living things that reproduce and thrive in optimal conditions, and the foods that we eat and how we serve these foods often create a prime environment for microbiological success stories. Bacteria, viruses, and parasites are microscopic organisms powerful enough to bring down whole populations; but with an understanding of how these organisms reproduce and thrive, perhaps we can better protect ourselves.

BACTERIA BASICS

Bacteria are everywhere; they are a normal and necessary component of the environment. Bacteria are found naturally in soil, water, and air. Animals and people carry bacteria on their skin and inside their bodies. Bacteria can also survive on inanimate objects that we use in the kitchen, such as cutting boards, knives, and sponges. There are as many as 40 different major groups of bacteria that are commonly found in food. Not all of the bacteria that are found in food cause disease, or are pathogenic, but many of them are. These include the bacteria that cause typhoid (*Salmonella*), kidney failure (*E. Coli* O157:H7), and paralysis (*Botulinum*).

Bacteria are classified in numerous ways. One of the principle means to group bacteria is to use a staining technique developed in the late 1800s by Hans Christian Gram, a Danish doctor. He used a purple-colored stain (crystal violet) while he was examining lung tissue under a microscope and noted that some of the bacteria retained the stain, while others did not. Those organisms that held the stain appeared purple under the microscope and those that did not retain the stain appeared reddish. It is still unclear what causes some bacteria to be capable of staining and others not, but speculation is that it is most likely related to the makeup of the organism's cell wall.

Even though all bacteria can not be categorized using Gram's staining method, it is usually the first step that disease detectives use to classify potential infectious agents. When the bacteria hold the stain, they are referred to as "Gram-positive," and when the stain does not effectively color the bacteria they are "Gram-negative." More than 100 years of Gram staining have given us pretty good data about where most known bacteria fit into these categories. For example, *Salmonella* is Gram-negative and *Staphylococcus* is Gram-positive.

Once the microbiologist has classified the bacteria according to Gram staining, the organisms are classified further according to their shape. There are three shapes of bacteria that can be observed under a microscope: coccus, rod, and spiral. Coccus-shaped bacteria are spherical or ovular in shape, rod bacteria are shaped like a cylinder, and spiral bacteria are shaped like a corkscrew. *Salmonella* is an example of a rod-shaped group of bacteria; *Staphylococcus* is an example of bacteria shaped like a sphere. One of the most common causes of human diarrhea, *Campylobacter*, is spiral in shape.

One of the other characteristics that help microbiologists identify bacteria is whether the organism needs oxygen to grow. If the bacteria can grow without oxygen, say in a can of green beans, they are considered "anaerobic." For example, the bacterium that causes botulism is anaerobic, it reproduces best without access to oxygen. Most bacteria need some oxygen to grow, so they are characterized on the basis of the level of oxygen that is most conducive to their growth.

Looking at bacteria under a microscope to see what they are shaped like and whether they can retain a stain may seem like primitive scientific approaches in these times of genetic sequencing and DNA analysis. But microbiology continues to be a dynamic science and new discoveries are constantly being made. By using basic universal techniques such as staining and identifying shapes, new pathogens can be classified into broad categories as they are discovered. Even as bacteria evolve into antibiotic-resistant strains, these basic techniques remain powerful tools in microbiology. At the same time, high-tech analysis is critical to helping us understand how some bacteria are changing and evolving.

Models of Evolution

Bacteria are the poster children for evolution. These microscopic organisms have demonstrated an energetic ability to change over time with their sole motivation being survival and reproduction. There is concrete evidence suggesting that bacteria are getting quite good at surviving many of the weapons in our environmental and public health arsenal. Our best weapons, antibiotics, have now even allied with some bacteria to produce stronger strains that threaten to sicken or kill more than ever before. An example of the public health threats from evolving bacteria began in early 2007 when the CDC uncovered a case of "extensively drug resistant tuberculosis" (XDR TB) in a young U.S. attorney.[7] This was such a significant case because the infected attorney had traveled by air to several countries outside of the United States.

While XDR TB is currently very rare, multidrug-resistant TB (MDR TB) is more common. TB is caused by bacteria that are quite stable in the environment, a fact that contributes to its transmissibility among people. When someone with TB coughs, he or she emits the bacteria into the air, where they can linger for several hours, depending on the ventilation system and the availability of ultraviolet light. For anyone who has ever traveled by airplane and experienced the ventilation conditions inside the passenger cabin, it should be easy to understand why there is so much concern about the travel habits of anyone traveling with any form of TB, let alone the XDR TB strain.

Regardless of the strain of TB, whether it is antibiotic-resistant or not, it is a disease that is not easy to treat. Treatment involves an extended period of antibiotic use, usually under the constant supervision of a health care professional. MDR TB has been proven to be resistant to the most common antibiotics and XDR TB has been proven resistant to the extremely powerful antibiotics that provide limited success with the MDR variety. The bacteria that cause TB are excellent examples of how microbiological pathogens evolve over time in order to ensure their long-term survival.

While TB is one example of evolutionary microbiology, another pathogen became a household word in 2007. MRSA or methicillin-resistant *Staphylococcus aureus* created a public health scare as the media were reporting outbreaks almost daily, many associated with schools. There were cases in which young people died from MRSA including a middle-school student in Ohio who died on December 20, 2007. In another case, a high school student in Virginia died from MRSA in the fall of 2007. Concerns over MRSA continued into 2008 and on January 2, 2008, the superintendent of a school district in New Jersey confirmed that one of his students was being treated for MRSA.

Although MRSA is usually a skin infection, it can lead to pneumonia, especially in relation to influenza. The CDC cautions public health professionals that healthy, young people can succumb to MRSA-induced pneumonia relatively quickly.[8] The emergence of MRSA in schools is somewhat puzzling to public health professionals because this pathogen is usually found in health care settings such as hospitals and nursing homes. However, the conditions of some of our schools creates an excellent environment to spread this pathogen because overcrowding is one of the leading factors in the transmission of MRSA.

MRSA is most likely to be spread from skin-to-skin contact, so athletes such as wrestlers and football players are likely targets for this disease. A wrestling program at a high school in northeast Ohio was temporarily shut down in the winter of 2007 because at least one of the team members had contracted MRSA. A high school in upstate New York was involved in a similar scare when one wrestler was diagnosed with MRSA, although the team was able to keep wrestling. Imagine a wrestler with MRSA having a bite to eat after a match, before washing his hands, and it is easy to see that the same pathogen that causes the skin condition can also be ingested and spread via food.

FATTOM and the "Curling Iron Waitress"

The TB and MRSA bacteria are spread in different ways, but both have evolved to be resistant to drugs that have traditionally killed them. TB is spread through the air and there is no evidence that it can be spread through the consumption of contaminated food. However, MRSA is an example of one of the many types of bacteria that can be spread through food. There are hundreds of other bacteria that can taint food in ways that lead to a variety of human health effects, the most common being gastrointestinal distress—that is, diarrhea and vomiting. There is no argument that bacteria are the leading cause of foodborne illness. These tiny organisms cause more human pain and suffering than almost anything else.

It is important that we understand how bacteria grow and thrive because this understanding can lead to better efforts to control their spread and changes in the way we manage the food in our own kitchens. Bacteria have needs, including a food source and ideal conditions under which to reproduce.

Environmental health professionals use the acronym "FATTOM" to re-member the important factors that contribute to bacterial growth. FAT-TOM stands for:

- Food
- Acidity
- Time
- Temperature
- Oxygen
- Moisture

Food

Bacteria generally grow best on foods that are high in protein. This is why we often associate food poisoning with meats, eggs, and dairy products. However, there are exceptions to the high protein rule, especially when the source of the bacteria is the food handler. For example, staph (*Staphylococcus*, or sometimes MRSA) is found on the skin and can be especially pathogenic around the sites of open wounds or burns. So, if a food service worker's hands are contaminated with staph bacteria, the bacteria can be transferred to any food source regardless of its protein content.

One case that illustrates how staph can contaminate non-protein-rich foods occurred at a small restaurant in a town in northeast Ohio.[9] This res-taurant was known for its fresh pies and was frequented by older people, both regular dining customers and those who just stopped in for pie and coffee. The local health department received some calls about people sick with gas-trointestinal illness and became concerned that there could be an outbreak when several cases stated that they had eaten at this small restaurant.

The environmental health professional, also known as a sanitarian, vis-ited the restaurant to take a look. He sat at the counter for several minutes watching the seasoned waitress serve food. The atmosphere was friendly and everybody seemed to be acquainted. The sanitarian watched as the waitress frequently scratched behind her ear and continued to serve food. At one point, he observed her slicing a piece of pie and using the hand she had been scratching with to slide the pie onto the plate. He approached the waitress, telling her that he noticed she seemed to be scratching and won-dered if she had a problem. She explained that she had burned herself with her curling iron and showed him a significant burn on the back of her neck that was showing signs of infection. Knowing that the staph bacteria love open wounds, it became clear pretty quickly that the waitress was the source of the bacteria that had made several people ill.

This case of bacteria being transferred from a food service worker to food is just one of many that occur on a regular basis. In most cases healthy people may never feel the ill effects of such poor food service practices, especially if they are consuming a ready-to-eat food such as a piece of pie. The problem with the "curling iron" waitress came to light because the clientele of the restaurant were largely elderly, who are more likely to become ill when exposed to even small numbers of pathogens. On the other hand, if the curling iron waitress had contaminated a high-protein food, such as lunch meat or cheese, and this food sat in conditions that promoted the growth of staph, even healthy people could have become ill.

Acidity

Acidity is measured by pH; the lower the pH value the more acidic the substance is. A neutral pH is 7.0 on a logarithmic scale of 1 to 14, and a pH over 7.0 is considered "alkaline" or basic. Bacteria do not like high acid (low pH) conditions, so foods like lemons with a pH of about 2.0 are less likely to serve as a host for bacterial growth than foods such as melons, which have a pH above 6.0. The acidity of citrus is one of the reasons why it is relatively safe to keep cut lemons and limes at room temperature for extended periods of time, such as in a bar. However, to ensure their safety, the lemons and limes should be washed, cut by someone wearing gloves or with clean hands, and using a clean knife.

In a food safety story with an interesting twist, the safety of cut limes, lemons, and other alcoholic beverage garnishes was the focus of news stories in late 2007. One New York City bar received a citation from the health department when the bartender did not use tongs or wear gloves when garnishing drinks. Food safety regulations in NYC do not allow bare hand contact with foods that will not be cooked prior to serving. There has never been a documented case of foodborne illness directly related to the lemons served in drinks, so this might have been overzealousness on the part of the health officer. However, bare hand contact with ready-to-eat foods is one of the leading ways in which bacteria are spread.

Time

Some bacteria take only seconds to reproduce and once reproduction begins it can be miraculously rapid. There are three phases in bacterial growth: (1) the lag phase; (2) the exponential phase; and (3) the stationary phase. The lag phase is the lazy time in which bacteria do not increase; they just hang out and adjust to the environment. After a certain amount of time and under the right conditions bacteria will begin to reproduce using binary fission, entering the exponential phase.

When a population of an organism grows exponentially, it can be thought of as a doubling or tripling of the base. So, if there were 1 million bacteria on a piece of chicken in the lag phase, as that chicken continues to sit at room temperature, reproduction can begin. Once bacteria start reproducing, their population could double every 10 seconds, so within just a few seconds there can be 2 million bacteria on the same piece of chicken. The more bacteria that infect a food source, the more likely a person can get sick from eating them.

There is not an unlimited supply of resources for bacteria to grow on that single piece of chicken. There will come a point in time when reproduction will slow and almost stop—this is the stationary phase for the bacteria. The stationary phase is basic population dynamics; any natural population that outgrows its resources will eventually stop reproducing and may even start dying off. One of the most effective ways to keep bacteria lazy and to stop them from entering the phase of exponential growth is by controlling temperature.

Temperature

Bacteria generally prefer a temperature around 70 degrees Fahrenheit to reproduce and thrive. Most bacteria will not leave their lazy lag phase if the temperature is too cold or too warm. This is the reason why refrigeration was such a major accomplishment in food safety. Most bacteria do not to grow well in an environment under 40 degrees, which is the temperature that your refrigerator should be maintained. Maintaining a high temperature is as important as maintaining a low temperature to keep food safe. When food is cooked and will be held before serving, such as on a buffet line, a temperature over 140 degrees is detrimental to bacterial growth. The 40-to-140 degree range is known as the food safety "danger zone." If a food contains bacteria and it remains in this danger zone for an extended period of time, exponential growth may occur, making the food unsafe to eat.

Think about a restaurant buffet as an example of using temperature to control bacterial growth. The salad bar area of the buffet should be kept at 40 degrees or below and the hot foods area should be at least 140 degrees or above in order to minimize bacterial reproduction. Simply stated, cold foods should be kept cold and hot foods should be kept hot. As with all of these rules of thumb there are exceptions, and there are some bacteria that actually enjoy colder temperatures and can grow best when they are being refrigerated in food.

When speaking about temperature–time relationships, time refers to how long a food stays in the danger zone. Some bacteria need only a few minutes under optimal temperatures to begin their exponential reproduction. However, the longer most bacteria remain at room temperature the more growth is likely to occur and the more dangerous the food may become. The time concept applies in situations like potlucks and picnics when people bring a dish to share and it sits at room temperature or higher for extended periods of time. The rule of thumb regarding time is that foods should not remain in the danger zone for more than two hours.

Oxygen

Remember that bacteria are living organisms, and many pathogenic bacteria are aerobic; that is, they need oxygen to survive. This is why proper canning techniques are a good way to minimize bacterial growth and why you can keep your canned soups in the cabinet rather than in the fridge even though they may contain high-protein foods. However, some extremely deadly bacteria thrive under anaerobic conditions. As noted previously, the bacteria that cause botulism are the best example of this. If these bacteria are present in the food during the canning process, sealing the can creates the optimal environment for reproduction. This is the reason why it is extremely important to sanitize all home canning equipment and to be wary of purchasing canned foods that are bulging, because this could be a sign that there has been some bacterial growth.

Although botulism is generally a disease that occurs on a small scale, being associated with home canning, occasionally there are larger outbreaks of the disease. One of the largest botulism outbreaks in the history of the United States occurred in Pontiac, Michigan in March 1975. There were 69 cases confirmed of botulism that were traced to hot sauce made from home-canned jalapeño peppers in a Mexican restaurant. Coincidently, the restaurant was located next door to St. Joseph's Mercy Hospital, so many of the victims were hospital employees.

A sanitarian involved with this outbreak recalls that this was in the days well before the Internet and cable network news, and by the time the Oakland County Health Division became aware of the situation and closed the eatery, it was past 7:00 P.M. and too late for the evening news. So a news bulletin went out over the radio by 11:00 P.M. explaining the situation and calling for others who were exhibiting symptoms to contact a health professional. The next day was chaos as members of the public who heard the reports and had eaten at the restaurant anytime during February and March appeared at hospitals and doctors' offices throughout southeast Michigan.

The bacteria that cause botulism are one of the most deadly substances known to humankind. It only takes a small amount of these bacteria to cause severe effects, including paralysis that could eventually lead to an inability to breathe on one's own. No one died in the Michigan outbreak, but three people were on respirators for more than six months. Interestingly, the hospital bought the adjacent property that was the site of the restaurant a few years later and the site is now a hospital parking garage.

Moisture

All living organisms need water to survive and bacteria are no exception. Generally, the less water there is in a food, the less likely bacteria are to reproduce. This is why it is safe to eat beef jerky and other dried meats, even though meat is generally one of the most hazardous foods. Drying meat can make it safe to eat and store at room temperature. Moisture is measured by the amount of water activity in foods and some foods such as cut melons, while not a high-protein food, have high water activity, which can create excellent conditions for bacteria to thrive. As a matter of fact, cut melons are considered a "potentially hazardous food" by the government, which means that you should take extra care in handling cantaloupe and watermelon, for example.

Controlling Bacteria

Of all of the microbiological organisms that can make us sick, we probably know the most about how to minimize our risks from exposure to bacteria. This is because we understand what bacteria need to survive and reproduce based on hundreds of years of research. The most effective way to eliminate bacterial contamination in food is to prevent it from getting in the food in the first place. This is especially challenging considering the nature of our food supply and the numerous ways in which food can become contaminated. By looking at the example of a hamburger as it is cooked in a restaurant, it should become clear that controlling bacteria is an endeavor that requires constant vigilance.

The first place that the hamburger can become contaminated is on the farm. Any time a population is packed into a confined space, the risk of disease transmission is high; this goes for people as well as animals. The largest beef suppliers raise thousands of cattle in very small spaces called concentrated animal feedlots. It is difficult to control the spread of infectious agents in these operations because of the proximity of the animals to one another. If one animal is sick, then it is possible to infect the entire group in a relatively efficient manner.

In order to protect their investment by minimizing the spread of infectious disease, many of these feedlot operations rely on preventive antibiotic use. A public health problem arises when the antibiotics used on animals are the same that people use to control human infections.[10] As we eat the meat that has trace levels of these antibiotics, we get just enough in our systems to kill the bacteria that are most susceptible, and leave the more antibiotic-resistant bacteria to reproduce without competition from the weaker strains. So, antibiotic use on farms may reduce the risk of acute bacterial infections in cattle, but it may lead to the spread of more virulent bacteria in the food chain, resulting in more dangerous infections in humans.[11]

Assuming that antibiotics do the trick and the cattle do not contain harmful bacteria, the trip to the slaughterhouse and the conditions at the slaughterhouse are the next stop in the potential chain of infection. Animals become stressed during the ride to the slaughterhouse and can defecate as a result of their stress. Feces can contain millions of bacteria (and viruses), therefore one sick animal can contaminate several animals during the ride to the slaughterhouse. Of course, the animals are cleaned before slaughter, but there is always the chance that some bacteria remain on the animals as they enter the meat processing plant.

The goal of meat processors is to produce as much meat in as little time as possible. This is one of the reasons that animal slaughtering is one of the most dangerous occupations in the United States.[12] The faster workers slaughter the animals, the more meat can be produced at the facility. Sometimes during slaughter the intestines of the animal can be accidentally cut, exposing all of the microbiologicals—both bad and good—to the meat-packing facility. If the animal is carrying a pathogenic strain of bacteria, such as *E. coli* O157:H7, these bacteria can contaminate the entire meat supply coming from the facility on that specific day. This is especially a problem for ground meat that is processed from scraps left after other prime cuts are completed. If one of the scraps contains the pathogen, it becomes mixed in with a batch of ground beef that could end up being shipped to numerous locations. This is the reason why it is unadvisable to eat an undercooked hamburger.

As the packaged ground beef leaves the processing facility, the next opportunity for bacterial growth begins. If, during the trip from the meat packaging plant to the wholesale or retail outlet, the product is not properly refrigerated, then any bacteria present can multiply. Remember the discussion about FATTOM and it is clear that ground beef is a good source of food for bacteria—it is a high-protein food. Bacterial growth can be controlled in ground beef by ensuring that the product stays out of the danger zone during transport and prior to placement for sale at a grocery store.

Once the ground beef is available at the meat counter for retail pur-chase, it essentially becomes your responsibility as the consumer to manage it safely. This includes getting it out of the danger zone that it enters as soon as you put it in your shopping cart until you arrive home and place it under refrigeration. It is up to the consumer to understand safe handling practices and the government requires a label on all meats to remind the consumer of this responsibility.

The final opportunity for harmful bacteria to increase in enough num-bers to make someone sick comes in the home. The major food mishan-dling factors in the home include improper cooking temperatures, leaving food in the danger zone for too long, and cross-contaminating other foods through inadequate sanitation. The result of consumer mishandling has led to some tragic foodborne illness cases in which children have been sickened and even died as a result of something their parent did in the kitchen. A recent case in Ohio in which a child died as a result of *E. coli* poisoning occurred when her parent did not realize that the raw ground beef he was using to make hamburgers came in contact with a bun. The child did not eat a hamburger, but she ate the contaminated bun.[13]

Bacteria are opportunistic organisms, and thinking about how the pro-duction of one hamburger creates numerous opportunities for them to be-come dangerous should be a wake-up call. But with so many hamburgers and other hazardous foods being consumed every day, why aren't we sick all the time? We are not all sick all the time, but we are sick a lot more than you might think. The CDC estimates that there are 76 million cases of food-borne illness in the United States every year, meaning that about one-third of the population suffers some sort of distress after eating contaminated food. One reason why we may not be alarmed about the bacterial contami-nation of our food supply is that we generally recover from what usually is a mild illness. However, recovering from viral causes of disease is often a little more difficult.

VIRUSES

Viruses are smaller organisms than bacteria and unlike bacteria, which are capable of multiplying on their own, viruses need a living host to survive and reproduce. Viruses are made up of genetic material wrapped in a coat of protein. They enter the unsuspecting host either by ingestion or inhalation and invade susceptible cells. Once inside the cell, viruses use the cell as their medium for growth.

When a virus successfully enters the body, a healthy host's immune sys-tem will attempt to kill it. However, if the host is unhealthy or its immune system is compromised, the virus might kill the host. This is not the ideal situation for a virus because if the host dies, so does the virus's ability to survive. This is why viruses are always looking for ways to infect additional hosts. In order to do this, they have become quite effective at hanging out on inanimate objects waiting for someone to invite them into their body. Viruses kill the host by either consuming healthy cells or by overtaxing the immune system while it tries to fight off the virus.

Viruses and Food

Viruses survive because they are constantly circulating in the environment. The viruses that we are most familiar with are those that are airborne, such as those that cause influenza (the flu) and the common cold. Some viruses can survive for long periods of time in the air or on inanimate objects, which are also known as "fomites." Viruses can be found in swimming pools, spas, and hot tubs, and on your computer keyboard. When a person inhales or ingests a virus, the virus searches for cells that would be the most conducive to its survival.

A major public health concern with viruses is in the emergence of new strains that have never before been identified. Emerging infectious diseases are generally those that have been discovered in the past 20 to 30 years and an example of one prominent emergent virus is the human immunodeficiency virus (HIV), which causes AIDS. Another emerging virus causes severe acute respiratory syndrome or SARS. West Nile virus was new to the United States in 1999, but it had been infecting people long before that in Africa, so it is not truly an emerging virus. However, West Nile virus in the United States is an excellent example of how viruses are really global infectious agents that can travel for long distances to infect populations far removed from areas where they are endemic.

Viruses that have been linked to food and caused illness most often are hepatitis, rotaviruses, and noroviruses. Although rotaviruses have been a major player in global outbreaks of diarrhea, many environmental health professionals believe that the major nonbacterial cause of foodborne illness might now be the group of viruses known as the noroviruses. The most disgusting feature of viral contamination of food is that it most often occurs because of poor sanitation, either personal or otherwise. Many of the viruses that cause foodborne illness live in the intestines of people and can only be spread to food from infected people who have not washed their hands after using the bathroom. This is known as the "fecal-oral" route of transmission.

Because viruses do not have the ability to reproduce in the absence of a host cell, the FATTOM criteria do not apply to them, with the exception of temperature control. Cooking food to proper temperatures is often an effective mechanism for killing viruses. However, the most important factor in preventing or minimizing the spread of viruses is good sanitation. Policing food service employees to ensure that proper hand washing is taking place is a tricky task and one that is not often a priority in food service. In addition, the use of gloves has probably created a false sense of security on the part of consumers.

One environmental health professional recalls the time he was inspecting a food service establishment and was impressed by the use of gloves by workers who were serving ready-to-eat foods. He was ready to give the restaurant a passing mark until he went into the bathroom. While in the bathroom, he observed a worker enter, remove his gloves and place them on the floor in the stall. When the worker was finished, he did not wash his hands, but put the same pair of gloves back on and returned to the floor. Glove use must be combined with good personal hygiene in order to be an effective prevention tool.

The most common viral stomach infection among children is caused by a group of viruses known as rotaviruses. These viruses are passed by the fecal-oral route, but usually on objects, not in food. Children in day care centers are especially susceptible during the winter months when indoor activities abound. According to the CDC, more than 55,000 children in the United States are hospitalized every year with this virus and more than 600,000 children die worldwide.[14] The CDC also estimates that virtually every child will have contracted illness from this group of viruses by the age of 4. The Food and Drug Administration (FDA) estimates that there are more than 3 million cases of this "stomach virus" in the United States every year.[15]

Most viruses are stable in the environment; this means that they can survive for long periods of time in water or food and even on inanimate objects. Imagine, for example, a childcare center in which one child is infected with a virus and is not skilled at personal hygiene yet. This child could carry the virus on his or her hands and then contaminate a wide array of toys and other objects that would be handled by other children. The only way to break the chain of infection is to apply sanitation techniques to kill the virus before it enters the body.

Controlling Viruses

Viruses cannot be treated with antibiotics, but this doesn't stop people from demanding antibiotics to treat them. The demand combined with the historical willingness of physicians to prescribe antibiotics for obvious viral infections, such as colds and influenza, have contributed to antibiotic resistance. The most effective way to control the spread of viruses is to take a preventive approach. The most effective preventive approaches are environmental health, personal hygiene, and immunization.

Environmental health measures to control the spread of viruses in food include clean water used for food preparation, good sanitation in the facility, and personal hygiene. The importance of ensuring clean water is emphasized by the fact that many viral foodborne outbreaks are associated with fish consumption. Shellfish are especially susceptible to viral contamination and there is evidence that oysters and clams provide substrates for viruses to grow to dangerous levels. The viruses get into the fish through poor water sanitation; that is, human and animal waste that taints the water in which the fish are being raised. This was one of the major concerns after Hurricane Katrina, when untreated human waste poured into the Gulf of Mexico.

Hurricane Katrina affected an area in the Gulf that supplies a significant amount of shrimp and oysters to U.S. consumers. Not only were entire fishing fleets damaged and lost in the storm, the pollution of the Gulf caused significant concerns over the ability of the fishing industry, especially oyster fisheries, to rebound.[16] Before Katrina, Louisiana was the second biggest producer of seafood in the United States, supplying about 25 percent of the seafood consumed in the country.

The fishing industry in Louisiana has yet to recover from the devastation, and some don't believe it ever will. From a food safety perspective, the waters in which the seafood is raised must be clean, and this will be a long-term process, so Louisiana fish may not be safe to eat for some time. This has translated into even more reliance on imported fish, especially shrimp, which may not be grown and harvested under the same conditions as American fish because of different regulatory approaches.

Because viruses continue to be such a significant cause of diarrhea, environmental health approaches might not be enough to control their spread.[17] There are currently effective vaccines for some viruses and these have been shown to be a cost-effective approach to controlling the disease. Hepatitis A is an example of a virus that can be transmitted to people from food, and there is a safe and effective vaccine for this virus. States that have required children to be vaccinated for hepatitis A have seen a dramatic decrease in the incidence of this disease.

PARASITES AND PRIONS

Other microscopic organisms that can contaminate food and cause illness include parasites and prions. Parasites create special challenges to safe food because they are sneaky. Food that is grown, processed, and prepared in the most sanitary conditions can become contaminated with parasites through the water supply. Some of the parasites that are in water are not killed using state-of-the-art disinfection techniques, so even water that is treated with chlorine may be the source of parasites.

Parasites need a food source to complete their life cycle and some parasites rely on more than one host to survive. Protozoan parasites produce a hearty cyst that can survive in the environment for extended periods of time, a factor that contributes to their spread via food and water. Microbiologists can only identify parasites by looking directly at them under a microscope. The good thing about parasites is that they are larger than bacteria, so they are more easily seen with the aid of good microscopy. The bad thing about parasites is that it is not possible to grow them in a laboratory. This means that the best way to determine if parasites are causing illness during an outbreak is to directly observe them in a sample, either food or stool.

The parasites that are most taxing to food safety in developed countries are the protozoa. Protozoan parasites that threaten the food supply mainly because of their presence in water include *Cryptosporidium*, *Giardia*, and *Cyclospora*. Unlike in developing countries, where parasitic worms pose greater challenges, developed countries are seeing outbreaks emerge in which protozoa are the culprits. One reason for this emergence is the demand for imported fresh produce, some of which comes from countries that may irrigate and wash the product with contaminated water. For example, *Cyclospora* is endemic in developing countries and people who are constantly exposed to this protozoan parasite develop immunity. However, when *Cyclospora* was imported from Guatemala with fresh berries, hundreds of people in the United States and Canada got sick.[18]

Aside from imports of fresh produce and fish, other factors that affect the emergence of parasitic diseases in developed countries include: (1) immigration; (2) aging populations that are more susceptible to infectious diseases; (3) demand for raw or undercooked foods; and (4) global warming.[19] In fact, global warming may create broad new food safety challenges and parasites are just one example. As water temperatures rise in areas that were usually cool, parasites that thrive in warmer waters could conceivably widen their range and become endemic in these regions.

The final microbe that is emerging as a possible threat to the food supply is known as a prion. Unlike viruses, which have a coating of protein surrounding genetic material, a prion is composed of protein only. It is smaller in size than viruses, and less is known about the microbiology of these organisms. Because of the scientific uncertainty and the link between prions and mad cow disease, public perception of their risk is high relative to some of the other microbes, and public perception of risk is often the major factor in driving governmental food safety policies and approaches.

ENVIRONMENTAL HEALTH AND FOOD SAFETY

Environmental health is a segment of the public health profession that addresses the relationship between environmental conditions and human health. It is the first line of defense against disease because its focus is on prevention. Although environmental health specialists, or sanitarians, are responsible for preventing diseases from numerous sources, ensuring food safety is one of their key job functions.

Environmental health specialists at the local level provide a community-based approach to controlling foodborne disease with comprehensive inspection programs. They conduct inspections at all facilities that serve food, from large restaurants to small vending carts that may be open only a few weeks per year. They are also responsible for inspecting institutions such as health care facilities and schools that provide meals to their highly susceptible clientele. Without these routine inspections, there would be a great deal more foodborne illness to contend with.

Unfortunately a major problem is that the environmental health workforce in the United States has been diminishing over the past 20 years. It is challenging to recruit people into the field because of the high academic expectations that include a significant background in the sciences, including microbiology, chemistry, and physics. Once graduated, entry-level environmental health professionals are greeted with many job offers, but the pay is quite low compared with other health professions. Environmental health practitioners can be classified into the group of professionals, such as teachers and nurses, who are indispensable to society but may never be paid what they are worth.

Professionals in the field of environmental health who are responsible for preventing and investigating outbreaks of foodborne illness must take a comprehensive approach. This means that they must have an understanding of food microbiology as well as be able to educate the public about food safety. In addition, the most effective environmental health personnel demonstrate the ability to solve problems, an ability that will guide them as they seek answers to why people are sick from eating food that was supposed to be safe.

Even if there was an unlimited supply of competent environmental health professionals, these people work in a political climate. This climate changes when administrations change, and if elected officials do not view public health as a priority, resources become scarce. Resource scarcity has been a major issue in recent years as public health, especially environmental health, has seen dramatic budgetary slashes and major shifting of resources from routine programs such as food safety inspections to more exotic programs such as bioterrorism. The result of this shift is starting to emerge as more people are succumbing to foodborne illness, and these illnesses are being associated with foods that are not the usual suspects.

NOTES

1. Matthew Philips, "They're Seeing Red over Greens," *Newsweek* 148 (October 2, 2006): 14.

2. Bernhard Schink, "Hans Günter Schlegel 80 Years Old," *Archives of Microbiology* 182 (2004): 103–4.

3. Hans G. Schlegel, "Continuing Opportunities for General Microbiology," *Archives of Microbiology* 182 (2004): 107.

4. Raymond W. Beck, *The Chronology of Microbiology in Historical Context* (Washington, DC: ASM Press, 2000).

5. The Galileo Project, "Fracastoro, Girolamo," http://galileo.rice.edu/Catalog/NewFiles/ fracstro.html.

6. Centers for Disease Control and Prevention (CDC), "Achievements in Public Health, 1900–1999: Safer and Healthier Foods," *Morbidity and Mortality Weekly Reports* 48, no. 40 (1999), http://www.cdc.gov/mmwr/preview/mmwrhtml/mm4840a1.htm.

7. CDC, "Extensively Drug-Resistant Tuberculosis," http://www.cdc.gov/tb/XDRTB/de fault.htm (accessed January 8, 2008).

8. CDC, "Severe Methicillin-Resistant *Staphylococcus aureus* Community-Acquired Pneumonia Associated with Influenza—Louisiana and Georgia, December 2006—January 2007," *Morbidity and Mortality Weekly Reports* 56, no. 14 (2007): 325–29.

9. All of the stories presented are actual accounts from practicing environmental health professionals during an online survey, November 2006.

10. Jennifer Weeks, "Factory Farms: Are They the Best Way to Feed the Nation?" *CQ Researcher* 17, no. 2 (2007), http://library.cqpress.com/cqresearcher/cqresrre2007011200.

11. Emanuel Goldman, "Antibiotic Abuse in Animal Agriculture: Exacerbating Drug Resistance in Human Pathogens," *Human and Ecological Risk Assessment* 10 (2004): 121–34.

12. Bureau of Labor Statistics, "Highest Incidence Rates of Total Nonfatal Occupational Injury and Illness Cases, Private Industry, 2005," http://www.bls.gov/iif/oshwc/osh/os/ostb1607. pdf.

13. Personal correspondence with former Food Safety Supervisor, Cuyahoga County Board of Health.

14. CDC, "Rotavirus," http://www.cdc.gov/rotavirus/ (accessed January 8, 2008).

15. U.S. FDA, "The Bad Bug Book," http://www.cfsan.fda.gov/~mow/chap33.html (accessed December 13, 2007).

16. Eugene H. Buck, "Hurricane Katrina Fishing and Aquaculture Industries—Damage and Recovery," *CRS Report for Congress* (September 7, 2005), http://www.fas.org/sgp/crs/misc/ RS22241.pdf.

17. Thea Kølsen Fischer et al., "Incidence and Cost of Rotavirus Hospitalizations in Denmark," *Emerging Infectious Disease* 13, no. 6 (2007), http://www.cdc.gov/eid/content/13/6/855.htm.

18. CDC, "Update—Outbreak of Cyclosporiasis United States and Canada, 1997," *Morbidity and Mortality Weekly Report* 46, no. 23 (1997): 521–23.

19. Ellin Doyle, *Foodborne Parasites: A Review of the Scientific Literature* (Madison, WI: UW: Food Research Institute, 2003), http://www.wisc.edu/fri/briefs/parasites.pdf.

— 2 —

Vegetables Can Be Hazardous to Your Health

At 6:03 P.M. on September 8, 2006, an independent microbiology laboratory contacted the Oregon State Health Department with news that they had identified four cases of foodborne illness that were caused by the same strain of *E. coli* O157:H7 bacteria. *E. coli* O157:H7 is a notifiable disease, meaning that whenever there are confirmed samples of it, the state public health authorities must be alerted. The purpose of requiring notification is to minimize the potential for a widespread outbreak. On this Friday evening in September, it was pure luck that there was someone still available at the state health department to take the call. A staff member recorded the call and decided that follow-up could wait until the following Monday.[1]

According to the Oregon state epidemiologist, on the following Monday, an intern was assigned to interview the people who were confirmed sick with *E. coli* so that they could begin the investigation into a common source of the illness. The intern did not complete the assignment on Monday and on Tuesday two additional sick people surfaced. It now appeared that Oregon might be in the midst of an outbreak, so it was critical that public health authorities focus their resources on this investigation. The six confirmed cases were interviewed using a standard questionnaire that asked them to remember everything they had eaten in at least the 72 hours before they got sick. By Wednesday morning, September 13, the Oregon Health Department determined that five out of the six sick people had eaten bagged spinach.

Maysville
Community & Technical College
Library

Rowan Campus-Morehead

At 1:14 p.m. on September 13, the Oregon Health Department sent an e-mail to the CDC with news that they had six cases of identical strains of *E. coli* O157:H7. At 1:27, the CDC e-mailed back that they were following similar cases in Wisconsin, New Mexico, and Utah, and that the strains all appeared to be identical. At 1:40, the Oregon Health Department replied, "We think it is bagged spinach." By 1:47, the CDC had organized a conference call with many of the affected states, and they verified that 13 out of the 14 sufferers in Oregon and Wisconsin had eaten bagged spinach.

Once public health officials agreed that bagged spinach was the most probable cause of the illnesses, the more difficult task began of identifying where the spinach came from and how it became contaminated in the first place. This investigation required quick and effective communication at all levels of government and between several states. Ultimately, an outbreak that could have spread to other states was contained with relatively minor public health impact. On the other hand, the economic impact to the bagged spinach industry and to bagged produce in general was much more significant than the actual public health effects.

While the 2006 spinach outbreak was an example of how the public health system can work when communication is optimal, it brings to light an important culprit in foodborne illness: produce. In terms of microbiological contamination, fresh produce is becoming one of the more dangerous foods that we eat. We are all reminded repeatedly to eat more fruits and vegetables, but sometimes doing so can be more hazardous than healthful.

THE PRODUCE PARADOX

Everybody knows that a healthy diet includes lots of fresh fruits and vegetables. This recommendation comes from both private health care professionals and public health officials. In general, Americans are eating more fruits and vegetables, but we are still not eating enough for optimal health according to health experts. However, as consumer demand rises for fresh produce, so does the need for more intensive agriculture and expanded imports. What's more, as agriculture intensifies and imports increase, the risk of contaminating produce with microbiological pathogens increases as well. Even with the potential risk of getting diarrhea from tainted produce increasing, public health professionals generally agree that the benefits of eating fruits and vegetables outweigh the risks of foodborne illness. This is evident in healthy eating guidelines prepared by the U.S. government.

The "Eat More Vegetables" Guidelines

The Center for Nutrition Policy and Promotion (CNPP) is housed in the U.S. Department of Agriculture (USDA) and is responsible for establishing dietary guidelines to promote healthy eating in the United States. American dietary guidelines were first developed in 1980 through a joint effort between the Department of Health and Human Services (DHHS) and USDA. The guidelines have a variety of purposes including offering scientifically based information on which to base food policy. The guidelines are also designed to educate the American public about nutrition. Because our understanding of nutrition is constantly changing, federal law requires the guidelines to be updated every five years.

The 2005 update of the guidelines notes that Americans are not consuming enough fruits and vegetables. This is despite the fact that, overall, our consumption of fresh fruits and vegetables has steadily increased in recent years. The 2005 guidelines recommend that Americans incorporate the following into a healthy diet:

- A sufficient amount of fruits and vegetables while staying within energy needs. Two cups of fruit and 2 ½ cups of vegetables per day are recommended for a 2,000-calorie intake, with higher or lower amounts depending on the calorie level
- A variety of fruits and vegetables each day. In particular, select from all five vegetable subgroups (dark green, orange, legumes, starchy vegetables, and other vegetables) several times a week[2]

These recommendations are based on scientific evidence that shows that people who eat the most fruits and vegetables are healthier than those who eat only small amounts or none at all. Some of the potential health benefits of eating vegetables are substantial. For example, eating dark green leafy vegetables, such as spinach, has been shown to reduce the risk of colorectal cancer.[3] Other benefits to eating a diet higher in fruits and vegetables include more control over weight, lower risk of heart disease, lower risk of developing diabetes and other chronic diseases, and even improvements in mood.

From Guidelines to Behaviors

Despite all that we know about the health benefits of eating fruits and vegetables, less than one-third of the U.S. adult population is eating two or more fruits every day, and only a little more than one-fourth eat three or more vegetables every day.[4] Women eat more fruits and vegetables than men, which may explain why, in many of the produce-related outbreaks, women comprise the majority of the cases. Understanding why we don't eat more fruits and vegetables is something that nutritionists, other health professionals, and researchers have been grappling with for years.

When it comes to consuming a healthy diet, with some exceptions, behavior change is required. Public health professionals are responsible for promoting changes in behavior in individuals and this is an extremely challenging task. We know that it takes more than just brochures, Web sites, and advertising campaigns to change behaviors. If it was possible to change behaviors by simply providing information, then no one would smoke cigarettes, everyone would wear seatbelts, and we would all eat more fruits and vegetables. Our best hope for promoting healthy lifestyles that include healthy eating patterns and exercise may be before children turn six years old. Research suggests that early patterns of diet and activity have been shown to last a lifetime.[5] Studies also show that as children move into adolescence, their fruit and vegetable consumption declines from year to year.[6]

Even though it is better to start with very young children, adolescents might not be a lost cause when it comes to improving nutrition. There have been some success stories in health-related behavior change interventions with adolescents. The most prominent is the campaign to cut tobacco use among teens. The strategy to curb teen tobacco use has employed a well-funded campaign that uses peer pressure in advertising to make smoking appear "uncool." It seems to have worked, as self-reported tobacco use among teens has been steadily declining. In 1995, more than 70 percent of teens had tried smoking and in 2005 this percentage shrank to just under 55 percent.[7]

While the fact that more than half of the teens surveyed say they had tried smoking is still too high, perhaps we can learn from the tobacco campaigns and employ similar strategies to promote fruit and vegetable consumption. Imagine, for example, similar ads to those designed to curb tobacco use modified to pressure teens to eat more apples and spinach. Teenage role models could be shown turning down one of their peers who is pressuring them to eat a super-size order of french fries and reaching for a bag of celery sticks instead.

A paradox exists because as we continue to promote increased consumption of produce, especially targeting children, we are also seeing more large-scale outbreaks of illness involving produce. If public health professionals are promoting increased consumption, they need to be sure that the product is safe.

A Safe Behavior?

While most environmental health professionals still view foods high in protein, such as meat and dairy, as major sources of foodborne illness, fresh produce is becoming a more important food safety issue. Fresh produce presents different challenges than meats and eggs, because we often consume these products raw. When we cook meat and follow temperature guidelines, dangerous microbial pathogens die. Of course, there are some meats, such as deli meats that are not cooked, and there have been well-documented outbreaks connected to their consumption. The same pathogens that contaminate meats, including *E. coli* and *Salmonella*, can contaminate produce.

When it comes to produce, we are encouraged to eat these with no or minimal preparation because raw vegetables and fruits contain more nutrients than canned or cooked ones. The hope is that most people wash their fruits and vegetables before they eat them, but washing may not be enough of a decontamination step. There are many factors that contribute to how produce can become infected with microbiological organisms. These factors include growing conditions in the country of origin, harvesting procedures, packaging and processing, transportation, and consumer preparation. By the time you pour dressing over the contents of that bag of salad, many people and machines have touched the greens, and any one of these could contribute to the spread of disease.

We know that outbreaks of illness associated with eating meats can lead to decreased consumer demand. One of the greatest behavioral change motivators is fear, and when people are afraid, they will take measures to avoid exposures. This was the case with mad cow disease, for example, when beef sales plummeted due to public fear of this exotic disease. The fear subsided however, and beef sales in the United States have recovered in part as a response to the high popularity of protein diets. It appears as if Americans are more afraid of societal backlash from being overweight than they are of the risk of contracting the human form of mad cow disease.

The role that public fear plays in meat consumption applies to produce as well. When there is a well-publicized outbreak that involves multiple states and cases, consumers may think twice before including spinach as part of their meal. Since there have been some widespread outbreaks in recent years, consumers are struggling more and more when deciding between the long-term health benefits that eating produce promises and the short-term risks from unsafe produce. If you are looking for an excuse to ignore the science documenting the benefits of fruit and vegetable consumption, you may have found it in the outbreaks associated with such items as raw sprouts and spinach.

THE SPROUT SITUATION

In addition to providing a great source of many essential nutrients, including protein, raw seed sprouts such as alfalfa, radish, and broccoli are also great sources of many microbiological pathogens, including *Salmonella* and *E. coli*. Sprouts are a healthy alternative to lettuce on sandwiches, they add a nice crunch to salads, and they are relatively inexpensive. However, because of the way sprouts are grown and processed, the potential for contamination by bacteria is high. Some of these bacteria can and have caused disease. Raw sprouts have been implicated in many outbreaks, and understanding the conditions under which sprouts are processed is helpful to understanding and minimizing their ability to spread pathogens.

In order to grow sprouts, it is necessary to create an environment in which the three factors that create optimal conditions for bacterial growth are available: moisture, warmth, and time. Recall that bacteria grow exponentially and, under the right conditions, a few bacteria can turn into millions of bacteria in a very short time period. Seeds used for sprouts can become contaminated at the farm or during germination, and studies have shown that some bacteria, such as *Salmonella*, can survive for months in seeds. So the bacteria wait in the seeds until they are offered prime conditions to reproduce, and the commercial sprouting process provides these prime conditions.

The first step in the sprouting process is to soak the seeds in water to begin germination. After soaking, the seeds are stored in a warm area with high humidity to speed up the growth from the seed to the sprout. For many of us the process of speeding up germination is reminiscent of elementary science class when we took a lima bean home and wrapped it in damp paper towels for a couple of days. I remember being amazed when the first green shoot sprouted from the bean.

In the case of producing sprouts for human consumption, if there are bacteria present in the seeds, they can begin to reproduce during the seed germination process. As the sprout develops, the bacteria will spread and contaminate the entire sprout. When someone makes a sandwich with sprouts he or she could be piling on bacteria with the turkey and cheese. Since the seeds are the most likely source of the microbial pathogens, it seems reasonable that the best place to minimize the risk that bacteria will be in the ready-to-eat sprout would be by treating the seed with disinfecting chemicals to eliminate the pathogen prior to sprouting. Treating seeds is one approach that has been recommended by environmental public health officials.

The Bad Seed

The process to make sprouts for people to eat has led the federal government to identify sprouts as a "special problem" in terms of food safety because growing conditions create the potential for exponential bacterial growth.[8] To address the challenges in ensuring the safety of sprouts, the FDA emphasized sprout management in the late 1990s and used an established federal advisory committee to help set sprout safety guidelines.

The National Advisory Committee on Microbiological Criteria for Foods (NACMCF) is an interagency committee that was established by federal mandate in 1988. As is the case with all federal advisory committees, NACMCF must comply with the Federal Advisory Committee Act (FACA).[9] FACA, which became law in 1972, requires all such committees to disband after a period of two years, unless they are renewed with a new committee charter. This is surely a political move so that advisory committees can be refreshed or terminated with each new Congress. The NACMCF has been rechartered every two years since its inception in 1988. The most recent charter is from August 2006, suggesting the importance and relevance of this committee to keeping the food supply safe.

NACMCF is made up of representatives from the U.S. Departments of Agriculture and Health and Human Services—specifically the FDA and CDC. As the committee name indicates, it serves to advise the federal food safety agencies about measures to reduce microbial contamination of the food supply. Their advice is to be based on the best available scientific information. In 1999, NACMCF produced a report that summarized the risks of raw seed sprouts, as well as potential steps to reduce these risks.[10]

Based on the NACMCF recommendations, the FDA issued guidance for sprout producers on October 27, 1999. As with most food safety initiatives, this guidance was not enforceable, so producers were not required to adhere to it. The FDA did encourage adoption when they emphasized that producers who followed the recommendations would also be in compliance with federal laws. The guidance included two important elements: sanitizing seeds and testing water used during the sprouting process for bacteria.

The NACMCF recommends treating seeds prior to sprouting with a combination of methods to eliminate pathogens, rather than relying solely on chemical treatment with a sanitizing agent. One such chemical method for sanitizing sprout seeds is by washing them with a chlorine solution. The NACMCF identifies the use of a 20,000 parts per million (ppm) formulation of calcium hypochlorite—that is, bleach—as one possible chemical treatment. This sounds like a lot of bleach, but it is actually equivalent to a 2 percent solution of bleach to water; similar to adding about 2.56 ounces of bleach to one gallon of water. The use of bleach has been somewhat controversial, as this practice may essentially pollute the seed with chlorine, and some are wary of the health effects of exposure to chlorine by-products.

In addition, there is continued research that calls into question the effectiveness of using chlorine as the sole sanitizing agent.[11]

Even though chlorine has widespread support in the sprout industry, it is interesting to note that the NACMCF did not specifically recommend bleach. Their report actually states: "Prior to sprouting, seeds should be subjected to one or more treatments that can effectively reduce or eliminate pathogenic bacteria (e.g. 20,000 ppm calcium hypochlorite)." The FDA issued guidelines with similar language, not specifically recommending bleach, but offering it as one alternative to chemical sanitation of seeds. It is well known that chlorine is not effective on microbiological organisms that are deep within seeds; rather it is most effective on surface organisms.

Despite the fact that the NACMCF recommends a variety of sanitizing methods, chlorine has become the predominant method for treating seeds because it is relatively inexpensive and has a history of being effective in killing microbial pathogens. However, chlorine is not a panacea, and its use could even lead to complacency on the part of producers. If we look at the way that we use sanitizing agents in our own homes, the complacency factor should be easy to understand. It has gotten increasingly difficult to purchase hand soap, dish soap, and even some facial tissues without antibacterial agents. Assuming that these products are selling well because of consumer demand, there has to be some general belief that antimicrobials will minimize the spread of infectious agents. This could lead some to take less care in hand washing because of the presence of antimicrobials in the soap. If food producers use a chemical sanitizer such as chlorine, there may be cases in which other sanitary precautions are less intensive or not monitored.

Almost immediately following the issuance of the guidelines for seed sanitation, researchers began evaluating the effectiveness of many of the recommended methods. This research was encouraged by the FDA and came from the NACMCF recommendation that the federal government expedite the review of other technologies for seed treatment. There are some other methods of sanitizing sprout seeds that are showing some promise and would minimize the use of chlorine-based products. One additional method, irradiation, appears to be effective in killing pathogens in seeds, but more research needs to be conducted to evaluate this method further.[12] Heat treatment in which seeds are essentially pasteurized much like dairy products also appears to be a promising alternative to chemical sanitization.[13]

In addition to treating seeds, another key element encouraged by the FDA in their guidance document is to enhance testing for pathogens in the water used to irrigate the seeds during sprouting. The FDA recognizes that even seeds that are treated with a chemical sanitizer may still contain pathogens. For this reason, testing the water that has been used to grow the seeds into sprouts may be an additional measure to identify the presence of microbes. Elevated levels of bacteria in the water are an indicator that the sprouts themselves might be contaminated.

Sprouts at Home

Many sprouts are packaged in plastic clamshell containers that make them appear as if they are ready-to-eat foods. This type of packaging encourages less vigilance on the part of the consumer and when the consumer takes the container home, it is less likely that sprouts will be washed in the same way an unpackaged head of lettuce or bunch of grapes would be. Now that we understand that seeds are the main source of bacteria in sprouts, washing sprouts might not be an effective technique in controlling the potential for foodborne illness anyway. In all probability, the best way to kill bacteria in sprouts is to cook them thoroughly, a method that is recommended by the federal government.

It is true that some of the sprouts that are implicated in foodborne outbreaks, such as mung bean sprouts, are used in such dishes as stir fries, so these are cooked. However, alfalfa and radish sprouts are sandwich condiments and are not typically cooked before eating. These types of raw sandwich sprouts have been implicated in most of the recorded outbreaks, which are commonly related to leafy sprouts such as alfalfa and clover. If you like to eat raw sprouts, it is probably a good idea to pay close attention to information related to outbreaks, otherwise you may be unwittingly increasing your risk of illness.

Sprouts were identified as a potential food safety issue in 1995. From 1996 through 2004, there were 27 known foodborne illness outbreaks associated with eating raw sprouts, and more than 1,633 people were ill. During this time, sprouts accounted for about 40 percent of the produce-related outbreaks and 20 percent of all foodborne outbreaks.[14] Most of the sick people consumed alfalfa sprouts and *E. coli* O157:H7 and several species of *Salmonella* were the most common pathogens linked to the illnesses.

The FDA was so concerned about sprout safety that they issued a consumer advisory in 1999 that cautioned the general public about eating sprouts. This was an unusual move because the FDA will generally only issue an advisory to especially susceptible populations such as the very old or young and those who might be most susceptible to infectious disease. In this instance, they decided that the risk of illness from consumption of raw sprouts was so great that even healthy people should not eat sprouts. The consumer advisory seemed to curtail outbreaks linked to raw leafy sprouts, but several new outbreaks emerged associated with eating bean sprouts. So, in 2002, the FDA updated its consumer advisory to caution the public about eating raw bean sprouts.

In 1998 and 2000 FDA personnel conducted inspections and field assessments at various sprouting facilities. In 1998, 57 percent of the facilities inspected were cited by the FDA as having unsanitary practices. In 2000, FDA expanded their inspections and included additional facilities, only to discover that almost three-fourths of the facilities received notification of unsanitary practices. The biggest problems with the facilities included unsanitary water and pests such as rodents and insects. In addition, personal hygiene of the workers and overall lack of cleanliness were noted at almost one-quarter of the facilities inspected.

In 2004, California environmental health officials inspected all of the sprout-growing facilities in the state. They used a standardized inspection survey to look for unsanitary conditions and found that 50 percent of the facilities were operating under conditions that could be contributing to contamination of the finished product. To put this in perspective, imagine yourself as the consumer picking up a package of raw sprouts and knowing that there is a 50 percent chance that the product was produced in a dirty facility infested with rodents—how might this knowledge affect your enjoyment of the product?

Another problem with sprouts is that many people don't even realize they are eating sprouts on fresh salads and sandwiches that they order in restaurants. This has prompted the FDA to refer to sprouts as "our stealth vehicle in foodborne outbreaks" because sometimes people consume them without evening knowing it. Besides, when people get diarrhea from eating a deli sandwich with sprouts on it, they are probably more likely to blame the meat than the "healthy" greens. On the other hand, blaming the healthy greens was rampant when one of the healthiest, spinach, created a nationwide panic because of *E. coli*.

DON'T EAT YOUR SPINACH

The foodborne outbreak associated with bagged spinach in 2006–7 should go on record as being one of the most important developments in food safety involving fresh fruits and vegetables. It was a national outbreak that involved a processed fresh product that is identified as one of the healthiest greens available. As the introductory portion of this chapter notes, it was quick work on the part of state public health agencies that caught the problem before it became a disastrous public health emergency. While the public health consequences have subsided, the economic consequences of this outbreak are still being felt by the bagged produce industry.

From Local to Global

Whenever there are two or more cases of the same food-associated illness, it is considered an outbreak. This may not seem like a high enough number because, after all, couldn't it just be a coincidence when just two people are unwell? However, from the public health perspective, if two people ate the same food and got sick, precautionary judgment suggests that it might just be the tip of the iceberg. In order for public health officials to be aware that there are sick people, someone has to contact them and report the symptoms. Most people do not think to call the health department and report that they have diarrhea or that they are vomiting, so the majority of foodborne illness goes undetected. This has led to the estimates often cited that 76 million Americans have foodborne illness every year—this is almost one-fourth of the entire population—and it is probably an underestimation.

Responding to foodborne illness has historically been a local public health issue; one restaurant, church supper, or relative makes a handful of people sick. Sometimes a physician will note several similar cases and contact the county or city health department. Other times the ill person will be so upset and convinced that a restaurant caused the problem that he or she will contact the local health department themselves. In any event, it is the local health department that often is the first to respond in the case of an outbreak.

Within local health departments, there are environmental health professionals who are trained to investigate disease outbreaks. These professionals use approaches in the science of epidemiology, which is the study of diseases in populations. Epidemiology is different from other types of disease research, such as medical science, because it focuses on populations such as a community rather than individual patients. The purpose of studying populations is to identify the most probable cause of disease and to recommend measures that prevent its spread to additional members of the public. Epidemiological methods include gathering as much data as possible from sick people and comparing the sick people with well people. In some instances the cause of the illnesses will be obvious but in many cases the culprit might never be determined.

Rapid application of epidemiology was the critical factor in curtailing the spinach outbreak. This outbreak is notable because it stands as an example of the effect that our food production practices can have on the public's health. This outbreak was also an excellent example of how foodborne disease has gone from local to global. The spinach was grown and processed in California and sold under several different brand names; the result was a national outbreak from a localized food source.

A major difficulty that is demonstrated by the spinach outbreak investigation was the possibility that there was product from several different farms in one bag. This makes tracing back—also known as "traceback" investigation—the source of the pathogen to one location extremely critical. To complicate matters further, the bacterial pathogen responsible for the illnesses was not one that is traditionally related to spinach. The pathogen is one that we have been familiar with for more than a hundred years and we understand because of the deaths of numerous people who ate undercooked hamburgers.

Discovering the Common Colon Bacteria

Theodore Escherich was a German pediatrician in the late 1800s and early 1900s. He was intensely interested in infant mortality and was very concerned about the incidence of diarrhea in children. He was an expert at recognizing types of bacteria under a microscope and wondered why more researchers weren't interested in the health of children. To get a better understanding of some childhood illness, he began examining fecal samples from children in the late 1880s. In the process, he identified 19 different types of bacteria in the stool of children. There was one bacterium that appeared over and over in the stool of children and he called it *Bacterium coli commune*, or the "common colon bacteria."

Although Escherich died young, at age 53, he had a legendary impact on pediatric science through his teaching and research. In 2007, it was suggested that he be identified as the first true pediatric infectious disease physician.[15] As is the case with many bacteria, after his death in 1911 the common coli bacterium was renamed *Escherichia coli* in his honor; now we call these bacteria *E. coli*.

Since Escherich's seminal work, there have been major advances in understanding these bacteria. As is the case with many microbiological organisms, the scientific study of *E. coli* is constantly evolving as advances in the science continue to identify new types of the bacteria. Generally, there are three categories of *E. coli* based on the illnesses they cause and where they are most commonly found inside animals. "Commensal" bacteria are those that are normal inhabitants of the intestines of animals and do not cause disease; they are even considered beneficial to digestion because they help in metabolism. The "diarrheal" category includes those *E. coli* bacteria that cause gastrointestinal illness, in some cases severe, bloody diarrhea. Finally, the "extraintestinal" group lives outside of the intestinal track and can cause infections in the bloodstream and urinary tract and other sites in the body.[16]

The *E. coli* bacteria are further categorized according to their antigen combinations. An antigen is a foreign substance in the body that causes an immune response. If antigens are present, it means that there is something trying to make the host sick. In the case of *E. coli*, there are two groups of antigens, the "O" and the "H." There are 174 O antigens and 53 H antigens currently known to microbiologists and these antigens have been assigned numbers.[17] Basically, the O number identifies the group that the bacteria belong to and the H number identifies a type within the group. When examining *E. coli*, scientists look for the combination of the O and H antigens and identify the bacteria accordingly. With this in mind there are numerous combinations, thus numerous varieties of *E. coli*, and 30 of the combinations are known to be responsible for diarrhea. The *E. coli* bacteria that cause diarrhea are also known as "enterobacteria" and can be furthered categorized in this group based on how they act in the intestines.

A distinguishing feature of *E. coli* is that it is not the bacteria themselves that cause illness. Rather, once they are ingested, the bacteria produce toxins that affect the lining of the intestines in different ways. For example, "enterotoxigenic" *E. coli*, also known as the cause of "traveler's diarrhea," produces a toxin that attaches to the intestines, but does not damage them to the point that they can not be repaired. Bacteria in this category are common in developing countries with poor drinking water sanitation. The diarrhea is usually watery and can lead to severe dehydration, but it is generally not fatal to healthy people, although young children may succumb to the resulting dehydration.

Another category of *E. coli* is the "enteropathogenic" group. This is the type of *E. coli* that Escherich discovered in the fecal samples he was examining from children with diarrhea. The toxin produced by this group can severely damage the intestines by causing cellular change. The changes lead to severe diarrhea that is an all too common cause of diarrheal death in children around the globe.

The "enterohemorraghic" *E. coli* group is perhaps the most frightening of the bacteria. This group damages the blood vessels in the intestines, a situation that can lead to bloody diarrhea. The toxin can also make its way into the kidneys, leading to one of the most serious outcomes of infection with the toxins produced from this group. If this occurs, the kidneys stop working, a condition known as hemolytic uremic syndrome or HUS. The only way to help the patient is to provide kidney dialysis. In some cases dialysis does not work and the victim dies from kidney failure.

Because *E. coli* is so common in the intestines of animals, when it comes to foodborne outbreaks, it is usually linked to eating meat products. In order for produce to contain these bacteria, the produce must be exposed to infected fecal matter at some point in its production. There are multiple scenarios for this type of contamination and several of these were possible reasons for the presence of the enterohemorraghic type of E. coli in bagged spinach.

Rare Spinach

Since the early 1990s, we have been warned not to eat rare hamburgers. This warning came in the wake of the devastating deaths of four children who had one thing in common: they had all eaten hamburgers. The problem was traced to a Jack in the Box restaurant in Washington state. When the smoke of the investigation cleared, more than 400 people were confirmed ill with an extremely dangerous pathogen that was still considered by health professionals as a relatively new cause of disease.

In 1982 the CDC, investigating an outbreak of severe bloody diarrhea, discovered a new strain of an old pathogen. This strain was identified as E. coli O157:H7. Although O157 and H7 were not new antigens, the combination of the two of them was never before documented. The common food source of the outbreak was undercooked hamburger; thus this strain became known as the "hamburger bacteria." That hamburger would be contaminated with E. coli bacteria was not that big of a surprise considering that mass production of ground beef could lead to the potential for fecal contamination of the meat. The surprise was that this was a diarrheal enterohemorraghic strain of the bacteria, causing severe bloody diarrhea.

Epidemiologic studies of E. coli O157:H7 led scientists to the conclusion that this pathogen can be found it both healthy and sick cattle, that it is a widespread problem in agriculture in the United States, and that calves are more susceptible than older cows to the pathogen.[18] Scientific evidence also suggests that very small doses of the bacteria can cause serious illness. Also problematic is that, since this pathogen produces a toxin, antibiotics cannot be used to treat the infection. As a matter of fact, antibiotics could create more of a health risk because of the potential for severe intestinal damage. So, this strain of the E. coli bacteria offered the absolute worst case scenario in terms of public health: a ubiquitous pathogen that is highly virulent and can produce an essentially untreatable illness.

Since its discovery in 1982, E. coli O157:H7 has been implicated in thousands of cases of diarrhea and hundreds of deaths. The most prominent source is ground beef, and the risk of meat products contaminated with these bacteria has led to numerous major recalls in recent years. For example, in June 2007, a California meat processing facility recalled almost 6 million pounds of fresh and frozen ground beef after 14 people in several western states were diagnosed with illness caused by the *E. coli* O157:H7 toxin. This ground beef was sold in numerous groceries including Albertson's and Wal-Mart.

The company that issued the recall, United Food Group, LLC, is a private company, so information about it is sketchy. It does not trade on the stock exchange, so there are no readily available records to examine. It is based in Los Angeles, California, and it processes and sells hamburger under the name "Moran's Ground Beef." Even though it is one of the larger meat processing facilities in the country, it is shrouded in the inaccessibility that a private company enjoys. The press coverage about the recall generally included verbatim notices from the USDA rather than company-generated warnings or evidence of concern. There was apparently a Web site set up for information about the recall, but by December 2007, the Web address no longer worked.

While we have been paying a considerable amount of attention to rare hamburger as the source of *E. coli*, the pathogen has been stealthily tainting produce. As discussed earlier, sprouts were a major concern because of their ability to be contaminated by the bacteria while in seed form. Spinach was just the most recent fresh produce casualty on this pathogen's radar. When one looks at how the situation with spinach was handled, there are some similarities between it and ground beef recalls. Like the ground beef recall in 2007, the company involved in the 2006 spinach recall was located in California and it processed and shipped spinach all over the country. One of the factors that likely contributed to the contamination of the spinach is the fact that despite being an "organic" product, the spinach was actually processed using intensive, large scale agriculture, in some ways more similar to beef farming than produce farming.

Factory Organic Spinach Farming

Natural Selection Foods was identified as the source of the contaminated spinach. This company is actually a network of organic farmers in the Salinas Valley in California. In 1995, Earthbound Farms partnered with Mission Ranches to create Natural Selection Foods. The partnership was expanded in 1999 when Tanimura & Antle, a major producer of fresh vegetables (not organic), and touted as a family farm, joined the group. According to their Web site, Earthbound consisted of about two and a half acres in 1984 and by 2007, Earthbound was growing produce on 37,000 acres, a monumental increase in both farming and produce processing.

When food production expands this rapidly, it becomes increasingly difficult to monitor food safety. Consider how much easier it was to keep both wild and domestic animals out of the crops when the farm was under three acres versus how difficult it would be to monitor 37,000 acres. Monitoring the growing fields is critical because *E. coli* lives in the intestines of animals, so it has to get into the produce either in the irrigation water or by direct contact. One of the leading theories explaining how the spinach became contaminated has to do with the access that feral pigs have to large-scale farm fields in some regions. If pigs defecated while the spinach was growing, it is possible that the spinach was either contaminated on the surface or that the bacteria could have been taken up by the seeds. As the sprout situation shows, seeds can contain enough bacteria to contaminate the entire plant.

In October and November 2006, state and local government researchers trapped and killed feral pigs near the ranches that were implicated in the spinach outbreak. They found *E. coli* O157:H7 in the intestines of the pigs, lending some proof to the theory of how the crop was contaminated. This was the first time that this pathogen was documented in feral pigs.[19] Even though the pathogen isolated from the pigs was the same strain as the one that caused the human illness, the researchers suggest that it is likely that additional factors were responsible for polluting the spinach.

Even if there were only small amounts of bacteria in the spinach, the way in which spinach and other bagged vegetables are packaged and sold to consumers offers excellent conditions for bacteria to begin their exponential growth phase. In order to keep the product appearing fresh, there is moisture inside of these bags and moisture availability is one of the important factors promoting bacterial growth. In the case of spinach, the bags traveled from California across the country. Transporting food this distance requires constant temperature monitoring to make sure that the food does not enter the temperature danger zone that promotes bacterial growth. If there was a problem with temperature during shipping, and bacteria was in the bags, they now had two excellent conditions, water and temperature, to start their exponential reproduction.

If the bacteria were on the surface of the spinach, they probably could be washed off if the consumer took the time to wash the produce. However, bagged salad mixes note that the contents are "triple washed," and this leads many consumers to think that no further washing is needed. The major reason that consumers spend so much extra money on prepared, bagged salads is the convenience. Washing the salad is something we would do to an ordinary head of lettuce or bunch of spinach, but bagged greens are considered ready-to-eat by many consumers.

The spinach outbreak and the seriousness of the sprout situation are just two examples of how important it is to be aware of problems with produce.

Many of the problems we have created as consumers who demand fresh fruits and vegetables all year regardless of where we live. Another problem is found in the lack of regulatory rigor when it comes to protecting the public from food safety threats. In general, the agencies in the U.S. government responsible for food safety have very little enforcement authority, although they do have the authority to make strong suggestions and recommendations to food producers.

PUBLIC PRODUCE POLICY

The government's central response to the spinach outbreak was to tell people not to eat spinach. They did not have the authority to mandate a recall; as with all food recalls, this was up to the spinach producers. There was also no information available about preventing the spread of disease that could be transmitted from person to person. For example, there were no announcements from the government about the importance of washing hands prior to eating produce. It has been suggested that if the government had initiated an educational campaign that encouraged more hand washing and other personal protective measures it might have had an impact on any secondary transmission that occurred.[20]

As with most of our government's approaches to preventing microbiological contamination of our food supply, the federal government has adopted several guidance documents to address the produce problem. These guidance documents are not laws; rather these are recommendations that encourage producers to follow procedures that will maximize safe food. Guidance implies "voluntary"; law implies "mandatory." Indeed, the public policy reaction to major food safety threats can best be characterized as asking industry to comply with specific standards, if they want to.

In order to address the real problems with foodborne illness associated with fresh produce, the FDA developed a Produce Safety Action Plan in 2004. This plan includes four key objectives:

1. To prevent contamination of fresh produce
2. To minimize public health impact when contamination occurs
3. To improve communication among producers, preparers, and consumers
4. To facilitate more research[21]

In 2007, the FDA issued the "Guide to Minimize Food Safety Hazards of Fresh-Cut Fruits and Vegetables." This was labeled "Draft Final" in March 2007, and noted on the cover was the phrase, "Contains Non-binding Recommendations."[22] The draft became final in February of 2008, and the statement about non-binding recommendations remains on the title page.

It seems as if the FDA is going to great lengths to reassure the produce industry that this document would not be a law that they would have to comply with. Rather, industry could choose to follow the guidelines voluntarily and there would be no penalty if they didn't because recommendations are not enforceable.

There are some very specific recommendations in the guidance, including an example of a sanitation schedule for a produce processing facility, and detailed protocols for environmental monitoring of air and water conditions. It is well known that tracing contaminated produce back to the source is often difficult, but the guidance suggests that that the processor "may" want to consider keeping better records. The guidance also suggests that the processor might want to consider some type of "coding system" to make products easier to trace back.

Of course there are other laws and regulations that produce processors must follow, but the tentative tone of this guidance must be frustrating to anyone who is concerned about whether they should cook their produce before they eat it, for example. It reads as if the FDA is almost afraid to offend the produce industry by making them do specific things that would actually minimize the risk of microbiological contamination in fresh fruits and vegetables. The word "recommend" is used at least 130 times in the guidance; the word "may" is used 61 times, most of which mean "might"; the word "encourage" is used five times; and the word "suggest" is used four times. Anybody reading the guidance without any understanding of the FDA could interpret the document as coming from an uncertain agency that has absolutely no ability to enforce regulations.

In addition to the general fresh fruit and vegetable safety guidance document, the FDA has been involved in several "initiatives" related to produce. In 2007, the FDA announced the multiyear "tomato safety initiative," a "leafy greens safety initiative," and a "lettuce safety initiative." The purpose of these initiatives is to examine the current procedures for processing these fresh products, conceivably so that additional "guidance" can be developed.

The safety of produce in the United States is chiefly in the hands of consumers. The federal government has guidance and initiatives targeted at farmers who grow and distribute produce, but none of these are mandatory or have the weight of law. When it comes to inspecting agriculture, the priority has always been on farms that raise animals for our food supply. Slaughterhouses, for example, are required to have a government inspector on site at all times, but be assured that this requirement does not mean that there will be no contamination of the meat supply, only that it will be minimized. Processing safe fresh produce has not received the same emphasis as meat processing and we are seeing the results of this now. At the same time that the government is urging us to eat more fruits and vegetables, there is no way that they can ensure that the produce we put on our plates is not teeming with microbiological pathogens.

Produce recalls continue regularly. In December 2007, 5,500 pounds of fresh basil that was imported from Mexico into California was recalled because of possible *Salmonella* contamination. *Salmonella* was also responsible for a nationwide recall of cut fresh cantaloupe in March 2008. Until the U.S. government has the authority to issue food recalls as it does when it comes to drugs and consumer products, we will have to wonder about the true magnitude of the food safety problem.

NOTES

1. Accounts of the Oregon outbreak come from presentations by the Oregon state epidemiologist and environmental public health officials from the CDC at the National Environmental Health Association annual meeting, Atlantic City, New Jersey, June 2007.

2. U.S. Department of Health and Human Services, *Dietary Guidelines for Americans,* http://www.health.gov/dietaryguidelines/.

3. Y. Park et al., "Fruit and Vegetable Intakes and Risk of Colorectal Cancer in the NIH–AARP Diet and Health Study," *American Journal of Epidemiology* 166 (2007): 170–80.

4. CDC, "Fruit and Vegetable Consumption Among Adults—United States, 2005," *Morbidity and Mortality Weekly Report* 56, no. 10 (2007), http://www.cdc.gov/mmwr/preview/mmwrhtml/mm5610a2.htm.

5. K. J. Campbell and K. D. Hesketh, "Strategies Which Aim to Positively Impact on Weight, Physical Activity, Diet and Sedentary Behaviours in Children from Zero to Five Years: A Systematic Review of the Literature," *Obesity Reviews* 8 (2007): 327–38.

6. N. I. Larson et al., "Trends in Adolescent Fruit and Vegetable Consumption, 1999–2004: Project EAT," *American Journal of Preventive Medicine* 32 (2007): 147–50.

7. CDC, "Youth Risk Behavioral Surveillance System," http://www.cdc.gov/HealthyYouth/yrbs/index.htm.

8. National Advisory Committee on Microbiological Criteria for Food (NACMCF), *Microbiological Safety Evaluation and Recommendations on Sprouted Seeds,* http://www.cfsan.fda.gov/~mow/sprouts2.html.

9. Federal Advisory Committee Act (Pub. L. 92–463, Sec. 1, Oct. 6, 1972, 86 Stat. 770.)

10. NACMCF, *Microbiological Safety Evaluation and Recommendations on Sprouted Seeds,* http://www.cfsan.fda.gov/~mow/sprouts2.html.

11. Megha Gandhi and Karl R. Matthews, "Efficacy of Chlorine and Calcinated Calcium Treatment of Alfalfa Seeds and Sprouts to Eliminate Salmonella," *International Journal of Food Microbiology* 87, no. 3 (2003): 301–7.

12. Sunil D. Saroj et al., "Effectiveness of Radiation Processing in Elimination of *Salmonella typhimurium* and *Listeria monocytogenes* from Sprouts," *Journal of Food Protection* 69, no. 8 (2006): 1858–64.

13. Haijing Hu, John J. Churey, and Randy W. Worobo, "Heat Treatments To Enhance the Safety of Mung Bean Seeds," *Journal of Food Protection* 67, no. 6 (2004): 1257–60.

14. Michelle A. Smith, Sprout Guidance, Next Steps, Public Meeting: Sprout Safety, College Park, MD, May 17, 2005. Available at http://www.cfsan.fda.gov/~dms/sprotran.html.

15. Stanford T. Shulman, Herbert C. Friedmann, and Ronald H. Sims, "Theodor Escherich: The First Pediatric Infectious Disease Physician?" *Clinical Infectious Diseases* 45, no. 8 (2007): 1025–29.

16. J. Michael Janda and Sharon L. Abbott, *The Enterobacteria* (Washington, DC: ASM Press, 2006).

17. Arun K. Bhunia, *Foodborne Microbial Pathogens: Mechanisms and Pathogenesis* (New York: Springer, 2008).

18. Gregory L. Armstrong, Jill Hollingsworth, and J. Glenn Morris, Jr., "Emerging Food-borne Pathogens: *E. coli* O157:H7 as a Model of the Entry of a New Pathogen into the Food Supply of the Developed World," *Epidemiologic Reviews* 18, no. 1 (1996): 29–51.

19. Michele T. Jay et al., "*Escherichia coli* O157:H7 in Feral Swine near Spinach Fields and Cattle, Central California Coast," *Emerging Infectious Disease Journal* (2007), http://www.cdc.gov/eid/content/13/12/1908.htm.

20. Edmund Y. W. Seto, Jeffrey A. Soller, and John M. Colford, Jr., "Strategies to Reduce Person-to-Person Transmission during Widespread *Escherichia coli* O157:H7 Outbreak," *Emerging Infectious Diseases* 13, no. 6 (2007), http://www.cdc.gov/eid/content/13/6/860.htm.

21. Center for Food Safety and Nutrition (CFSAN), *Produce Safety from Production to Consumption: 2004 Action Plan to Minimize Foodborne Illness Associated with Fresh Produce Consumption*, http://www.cfsan.fda.gov/~dms/prodpla2.html.

22. FDA, *Guide to Minimize Microbial Food Safety Hazards of Fresh-cut Fruits and Vegetables*, http://www.cfsan.fda.gov/~dms/prodgui3.html.

— 3 —

Rotten Eggs and Peanut Butter

Remember, when you were a kid, how great raw cookie dough tasted? The thick, sugary concoction was motivation enough to bake cookies and forget about waiting for them to come out of the oven. Many of us probably have fond memories of baking with our families and barely having enough dough left to put on cookie sheets for baking. Times, and eggs, have changed, and as I bake with my own children today, they are not allowed to sample the raw dough. I am afraid that they will get diarrhea from a bacteria that is lurking inside a large percentage of eggs, and that their memories of baking will not be as fond as mine.

Salmonella is a bacterial pathogen that microbiologists and environmental health scientists have known about for more than one hundred years, but it wasn't until relatively recently that it has been identified as one of the major contributors to foodborne illness. *Salmonella* is most often connected with eggs and other poultry products, but it is becoming a major concern in many other foods, from peanut butter to frozen pot pies.

SALMONELLA MICROBIOLOGY

Salmonella is a somewhat confusing pathogen to understand mainly because of its taxonomy. It is part of a large family of bacteria known as "enterobacteria." These bacteria are Gram-negative, meaning that they do not retain color after being stained in the laboratory. They are also considered one of the most important groups of bacteria because of their ability to cause human disease. In addition to foodborne infections that result in diarrhea and other gastrointestinal distress, they have been identified as the cause of blood infections, respiratory illnesses, urinary tract infections, and wound infections. This is important because these bacteria live in the intestines of humans and animals, so their ability to cause these so-called extraintestinal infections makes the control of enterobacteria one of the most important environmental health priorities we face.

Infections of the blood, the respiratory and urinary tracts, and surgery sites are increasing in the human population and enterobacteria are the leading cause of this trend. Of course one of the reasons for this increase in disease is related to our expanding life expectancy, which leads to an aging population that may be more susceptible to illness. In addition, as people age and become reliant on assisted living or long-term care, they often require invasive procedures such as catheterization that can contribute to the spread of these pathogens.[1] This is one reason why the elderly have the highest rate of urinary tract infections of all populations. Gram-negative bacteria are the likely cause of more than 40 percent of these infections, with E. coli being the leader of the pack.[2]

When investigating the cause of infectious disease outbreaks, appropriately naming and classifying the offending microorganisms is extremely important for a number of reasons. In terms of foodborne illness, using accepted, universal terminology for the microorganisms may be crucial to identifying the source of the pathogens and the number of people who have been affected, and to stopping the spread of an outbreak. Investigating illness caused by Salmonella bacteria offers an excellent example of the importance of terminology.

Salmonella is not a single bacterium, rather it consists of two species in the genus Salmonella: enterica and bongori. Grouping the bacteria into these two species has been somewhat controversial and it wasn't until 2005 that this categorization was accepted by an international commission responsible for suggesting changes to the International Code of Nomenclature of Bacteria.[3] This code has been in place since the 1940s and includes principles for naming microorganisms as they are discovered.[4] The code is constantly updated because microbiology is such a dynamic science.

Within the two Salmonella species, there are several subspecies. In the Salmonella enterica group, there are six subspecies: enterica or group I; salamae or group II; arizonae or group IIIa; diarizonae or group IIIb; houtenae or group IV; and indica or group VI. There is currently no group V subspecies. These six subspecies are found throughout the environment, but some of them are more commonly associated with food than others. Understanding these groupings will be important as the contemporary outbreaks of *Salmonella* are discussed below.

To further categorize the subspecies and narrow the identification of *Salmonella*, within these subspecies there are numerous different types, also known as "serovars" or "serotypes." According to the CDC, there were at least 2,541 serotypes of *Salmonella* as of 2002.[5] New serotypes are still being discovered and as these bacteria evolve to become increasingly resistant to antibiotics, we may see additional serotypes within the next 10 years. Serotypes are not italicized when they are written; they are capitalized.

The majority of foodborne illness caused by *Salmonella* is caused by the *enterica* subspecies. Three main serotypes in this subspecies that are most commonly found during outbreaks are: (1) Typhimurium, (2) Enteritidis, and (3) Newport. As new serotypes of *Salmonella* are identified they are often named after the location of their discovery. For example, one of the newer strains, *Salmonella* Tennessee (discussed below), was first identified in Tennessee. This serotype could also be written as *Salmonella enterica* Tennessee.

Classifying the *Salmonella* genus recently created a controversy among microbiologists as a decision was made to use the name *S. enterica* as the standard for identifying different strains of the bacteria.[6] During an outbreak of salmonellosis, you might see something like, "*Salmonella* serotype Enteritidis was identified as the cause of the illness." This can be translated to mean that the serotype Enteritidis in the *enterica* subspecies was identified as the pathogen. All of this discussion and controversy surrounding the nomenclature of *Salmonella* emphasizes the fact that discoveries are still being made about the nature of these bacteria and it is likely that we will continue to find new strains for some time to come.

Of all the serotypes of *Salmonella enterica*, Typhimuirum and Enteritidis have been identified most often as the cause of human illness. In 2005, Typhimurium and Enteritidis were identified in more than 37 percent of the human cases of salmonellosis.[7] However, some more recent outbreaks have involved large numbers of people and rare forms of *Salmonella* have been identified as the culprits.

SCANDALOUS *SALMONELLA*

Salmonella has an interesting history complete with backstabbing scientists, an iconic disease-spreading cook, and evidence of its contribution to the fall of an ancient empire. Throughout its history, the serotype of the bacteria that causes typhoid fever has been the most prominent.

Backstabbing Science

Salmonella is a group of bacteria that was named after Dr. Daniel E. Salmon. Dr. Salmon was a well-known veterinarian who studied infectious diseases in domesticated animals, with a major focus on tuberculosis in cattle. In 1884, he was the founding director of the U.S. Department of Agriculture's Bureau of Animal Industry.[8] The initial responsibility of this bureau was to study disease in animals and to determine if these diseases could be transmitted to humans. According to the National Archives, the Bureau of Animal Industry was the segment of the Department of Agriculture that "conducted scientific investigations and administered statutes and regulations to protect the public from infected or diseased meat products, eradicate animal diseases, and improve livestock quality."[9]

During his professional career, Salmon made some remarkable contributions to animal and public health. He is credited with being one of the first researchers to confirm that animals can indeed spread disease to humans.[10] However, this acknowledgment is somewhat clouded by a controversy surrounding his relationship with Dr. Theobald Smith. Daniel Salmon graduated from Cornell University in 1872 with a bachelor's degree in veterinary medicine. He never earned a doctorate; rather he was awarded an honorary doctorate in veterinary medicine from Cornell in 1876. When he was appointed to his job in the Department of Agriculture, he sought help from Cornell faculty to select a laboratory assistant; Theobald Smith came highly recommended.

Dr. Smith, who is now regarded as one of the most important researchers in the field of medicine, had an MD from Albany Medical College and was at first honored to be offered work at the Department of Agriculture under Salmon. This honor soon turned into frustration as Salmon repeatedly took credit for much of Smith's work. Accounts from Smith's diary, as reprinted in his biography, show an increasingly aggravated man as Salmon would make presentations at national conferences and submit reports based solely on Smith's work, but not even mention Smith's name.[11]

By most accounts it was Dr. Smith who first isolated the *Salmonella* bacteria, but Salmon took full credit for the discovery. This is not unusual in the field of research even today, as the supervisors of young researchers often identify themselves as the pioneers or leaders in their respective fields. This occurs routinely when senior researchers place their names on articles that are published to document important scientific discoveries. What is a little unusual in this case is that the bacterium that Smith identified was eventually named after Salmon, thereby memorializing Salmon's usurpation of Smith's discovery. Smith eventually grew to despise Salmon and felt vindicated when Salmon's credentials were discredited on the witness stand during a trial about arsenic pollution in Butte, Montana.

Having a bacterial pathogen that causes diarrhea and stomach cramps named after you is probably not something many of us aspire to, so perhaps Dr. Smith was not bothered by the lack of credit at the time. As a matter of fact, Dr. Smith went on to become one of the most influential researchers who ever studied the transmission of disease from animals to humans. For example, he is credited with identifying ticks as vectors of disease, a finding that has great implications today for our understanding diseases such as Lyme disease and Rocky Mountain spotted fever.

History has been kind to Dr. Smith, and most accounts of the identification of *Salmonella* note that this was actually his discovery not Salmon's. It is more difficult to find biographical information about Salmon than it is about Smith, another indicator of Smith's prominence in science. The New Jersey branch of the American Society of Microbiology even calls itself "The Theobald Smith Society." Presumably because of his contribution to our understanding infectious disease, when Dr. Smith died in 1935, his obituary stated that "all men are Dr. Smith's debtors."[12]

End of the Golden Age

Even though *Salmonella* was discovered by Smith in the late 1800s and named after Salmon at this time, it may actually be an ancient bacterium dating back to 500 B.C. It could even have been responsible for the Plague of Athens that contributed to the fall of the Greek city. The plague occurred in Greece during a time that was known as the "Golden Age." It was a period in history that brought some of the most influential architecture, philosophy, religion, art, and literature ever recorded. During the Golden Age, Socrates lived in Greece, the Parthenon was built, and a fierce competition surfaced between the two major cities: Athens and Sparta. The result of the competition was the Peloponnesian War that began in 431 B.C. and ended in 404 B.C.

Recent research suggests that *Salmonella* may have been the pathogen responsible for the Plague of Athens from 430 to 426 B.C.[13] In the mid-1990s, Greek researchers were able to take dental material from skeletons found in a mass grave in Athens, Greece. They dated the grave back to the Plague of Athens and identified the remains as victims of the plague. The researchers used DNA analysis to search for six possible pathogens including anthrax, tuberculosis, and cowpox. The only genetic material that they were able to confirm in all of the samples corresponded to *Salmonella* Typhi, leading them to suggest that this may have been the cause of the plague. *Salmonella Typhi* is the cause of typhoid fever.

Historians rely on the records of Thucydides, who was an Athenian aristocrat, for accounts of the Peloponnesian War. He made direct observations of the war and the illness that was gripping Athens during this time. Throughout the war, people crowded into Athens, creating excellent conditions and opportunities for disease transmission. Today, environmental health professionals understand that one of the leading contributors to the spread of infectious disease is overcrowding in unsanitary conditions, and this is likely to have been the case during this time.

According to Thucydides, Athenians first became ill during the summer of 430 B.C. He took detailed notes and recorded many observations all through the war and noted that illness broke out twice more in 429 and 427 B.C. Thucydides described the outbreaks as follows:

If any man were sick before, his disease turned to this; if not, yet suddenly, without any apparent cause preceding and being in perfect health, they were taken first with an extreme ache in their heads, redness and inflammation of the eyes; and then inwardly, their throats and tongues grew presently bloody and their breath noisome and unsavoury. Upon this followed a sneezing and hoarseness, and not long after the pain, together with a mighty cough, came down into the breast. And when once it was settled in the stomach, it caused vomit; and with great torment came up all manner of bilious purgation that physicians ever named...Their bodies outwardly to the touch were neither very hot nor pale but reddish, livid, and beflowered with little pimples and whelks, but so burned inwardly as not to endure any the lightest clothes or linen garment to be upon them nor anything but mere nakedness, but rather most willingly to have cast themselves into the cold water.[14]

What Thucydides seems to be saying is that people who were already sick, or those whom we would call immunocompromised today, would subsequently display the symptoms of this new illness. Furthermore, healthy people were struck with illness in an acute way, appearing healthy one minute and sick the next. He observed headaches, fever, diarrhea, vomiting, and a strange rash on people who were sick.

According to the online source Medline, the symptoms for typhoid fever are "generalized and include fever, malaise and abdominal pain. As the disease progresses, the fever becomes higher (greater than 103 degrees Fahrenheit), and diarrhea becomes prominent. Weakness, profound fatigue, delirium, and an acutely ill appearance develop. A rash, characteristic only of typhoid and called "rose spots," appears in some cases of typhoid. Rose spots are small (1/4 inch) red spots that appear most often on the abdomen and chest. Typically, children have milder disease and fewer complications than adults."[15]

The symptoms described by Thucydides and Medline are similar enough to support the likelihood that *Salmonella* Typhi could have caused the plague. Modern DNA analysis provides stronger evidence that this was the case. The conditions described by Thucydides also point to an environment in which the spread of typhoid could be rampant. One notable death during the plague was Pericles, the democratic leader of Athens, who succumbed to the plague one year into the Peloponnesian War. His death was significant enough that history might have been quite different if this infectious disease had not been running rampant throughout Athens.

The DNA analysis is not a "slam dunk" when it comes to blaming *Salmonella* for the "end of the Golden Age" in Athens. While DNA analysis is a reliable method, it is possible that the pathogen is actually a "modern" one that found its way into the teeth through the surrounding soil.[16] However, Thucydides' accounts suggest that the plague was isolated to humans, and typhoid fever is one serotype of *Salmonella* that only affects humans, it is not found in other animals. The debate about what caused the Plague of Athens will likely continue and it will be interesting to see additional research on the subject.

Cooking up a Wealthy Diarrhea

While we may never know for sure if Typhi caused the Plague of Athens, we do know that it was responsible for the most infamous case of *Salmonella* food poisoning in the United States. This dates back to the early 1900s with the case of Mary Mallon. Mallon was a cook for many wealthy families in New York and unknowingly was a carrier of *Salmonella* Typhi. A chronology of Mary Mallon's activities shows that she was the likely cause of the illness of many people.[17] However, she was specifically linked to causing at least 47 people to become ill, and at least three of these people died from their illness.

In the early 1900s, Oyster Bay, New York, was a popular vacation spot for the rich and influential. President Theodore Roosevelt owned a home in the community and spent at least part of his summers there; he died and was buried in Oyster Bay in 1919. Mary Mallon was hired as a cook for one of the families vacationing in the community. In 1906, six of the 11 people in the home where she was working were diagnosed with typhoid. At this time in history, it was already known that typhoid was caused by bacteria.

Dr. George Soper was a civil engineer, and he was hired to find the source of the bacteria that made the family sick. He focused first on the drinking water on the property because he knew that typhoid could contaminate the water supply. He found no evidence of bacteria in the water. Because it is possible for these bacteria to remain in the environment for extended periods of time, Soper researched the history of the house. The ill family who was renting for the summer and Soper hypothesized that the bacteria were somewhere in the house, brought there by a former tenant. This approach turned into a dead end as Soper found no evidence of anyone who had stayed at the house previously being ill.

Soper then turned to investigating food as the source of the bacteria. He first suspected it might be clams that were harvested from the bay. If the clams were harvested from polluted water, it is likely that they could be contaminated with bacteria. However, no one in the house had eaten clams. Finally, he discovered that the family had changed cooks about two weeks before the first person became ill. He approached this new cook, Mary Mallon, and asked for her cooperation with the investigation; she refused. Accounts of her refusal suggest that she was violent in her reaction to Soper and subsequently disappeared from the home.[18]

Since Ms. Mallon refused to cooperate with the investigation, Soper was forced to act as an amateur detective to try to link the cook with the spread of disease. He researched previous places she had worked and discovered at least four other outbreaks of typhoid in places where Mary had worked. The interesting thing was that Mary never became ill herself.

Mary Mallon was a carrier of the bacteria that causes typhoid fever although she never had symptoms herself. The bacteria were in her stomach and she said herself that she rarely washed her hands after using the bathroom. So the ultimate cause of her spreading the bacteria was likely her own poor personal hygiene. Mary Mallon was eventually caught, and her stool tested positive for *Salmonella* Typhi; she was subsequently quarantined, and history remembers her as "Typhoid Mary."

Salmonella Typhi only lives in humans; it is not found in animals. So it is not a pathogen that can be spread from improperly cooked food such as an undercooked egg. It is spread by bare-hand contact with ready-to-eat foods or by other human contamination during food preparation. This reality is unpleasant to ponder. As with some of the other "fecal-oral" food pathogens, if you have contracted *Salmonella* Typhi, it is likely that you contracted it from ingesting fecal matter from someone who touched your food, or from water that was not treated to kill these bacteria.

SALMONELLA FEVER

When water is the mode of transmission for *Salmonella* Typhi it is evidence that the water that has not been cleaned or treated adequately. Untreated water may contain raw sewage and all of the pathogens that are found in human waste. Although typhoid is rare in developed countries with good water sanitation, it is more common in nations with primitive or no water treatment capabilities. The CDC estimates that almost 75 percent of the American cases of typhoid fever occur in people who have traveled abroad.[19] Even though the number of cases of typhoid in the United States has remained relatively stable for some time, averaging about 400 per year, the likelihood that the illness is related to travel has increased substantially since 1975.[20] There is evidence that even a short-term stay in a country with endemic typhoid could put a traveler at risk.

On the global scale, the typhoid picture is much more dramatic. According to the CDC, there are as many as 22 million cases of typhoid fever and nearly 200,000 deaths from the illness across the globe every year. Areas in the world that put travelers at the greatest risk of contracting the disease include South Asia, Africa, the Caribbean, and Central and South America.[21] The World Health Organization (WHO) estimations are a little more robust than the CDC's and they calculate that there are somewhere between 16 and 33 million cases of typhoid fever every year and as many as 500,000 to 600,000 deaths.[22] Death from typhoid is the result of diarrhea that leads to dehydration. Treating diarrhea requires taking in excess fluids, and when the only fluids available contain the pathogen that caused the diarrhea, the outcome could be deadly.

It is possible to be vaccinated against typhoid and the CDC recommends a vaccine for people who will be traveling to South Asia in particular, because it is common to see antibiotic-resistant strains of *Salmonella* Typhi in this region. Existing vaccines for typhoid fever have been proven effective, but they are not currently available for children under the age of two, even though this age group appears to be highly susceptible to the illness.[23] While vaccination is a good preventive strategy, it implies that areas where typhoid is endemic are able to afford large-scale vaccination; this simply is not the case. Typhoid is a symptom of poverty and an inadequate environmental health infrastructure. There is no reason to believe that vaccination is the panacea that will solve the worldwide typhoid problem unless poverty is eradicated or the vaccine is available free.

The nature of typhoid contributes to its impact on populations that are unexpectedly forced to live in crowded areas with poor sanitation. This is one reason why there is concern about outbreaks of the disease during natural disasters such as floods, and human-made disasters such as war. There is evidence, for example, that typhoid was imported into Croatia from Bosnia and Herzegovina during the conflict from 1991 to 1995. Prior to 1992, there were no cases of typhoid on record in Croatia, but from 1992 to 1998, 45 cases were identified.[24]

Although there is currently no documented evidence readily available of an outbreak of typhoid in Iraq, this war has led to the disruption of basic public health services. These include vaccination programs and environmental health infrastructure, such as water treatment. The combination of the lack of prevention and the disruption in sanitation creates ideal conditions for a public health disaster to occur in Iraq.[25]

Natural disasters in developing countries, such as the 2007 monsoon rains in India and Bangladesh, are of great concern with respect to the spread of typhoid due to the lack of good water sanitation. There is emerging apprehension that climate change will contribute to more extreme global weather conditions, leading to more natural disasters that could further create circumstances favoring the spread of typhoid. To date, people living in the midst of natural disasters in developed countries have largely been spared the impact of typhoid; one extreme disaster in the United States in 2005 stands as an example of this.

During Hurricane Katrina, some health experts, but mostly the media, warned of a risk from typhoid. However there were no reported cases of typhoid linked specifically to the environmental conditions immediately after Hurricane Katrina, and the CDC did not even recommend vaccination for typhoid during this event. The CDC was more concerned about hepatitis and tetanus during Katrina and recommended vaccination for these two illnesses, especially for health care workers and first responders. There were cases of gastrointestinal distress during the aftermath of Katrina, but these were likely caused by viruses or other bacteria that are endemic to the area.

Although typhoid fever has historically been treatable with antibiotics, there are new worries that this pathogen is becoming increasingly resistant to some of the most powerful antibiotics available.[26] The most effective way to control the spread of typhoid is through a combination of vaccination, antibiotic treatment, and sound environmental health. These three strategies require resources that are often not available to the most susceptible populations, making typhoid an issue of equity as well as health. The fact that typhoid is not uncommon in developing countries, and that it did not surface as a major public health threat during the greatest natural disasters in contemporary U.S. history, underscores the role that poverty plays in the incidence of this disease.

MORE COMMON THAN TYPHOID

There are other strains of *Salmonella* that do not specifically target poor populations. The illnesses caused by these strains are largely the result of ingesting contaminated food, something that richer nations do more frequently than poorer nations. Typhoid fever is perhaps the most notorious serotype of *Salmonella*, but it is not the strain that causes the most foodborne illness in developed countries. As noted previously, there are three other serotypes that have been major contributors to foodborne illness. These serotypes have found their way into commonly consumed items such as peanut butter and pot pies.

Salmonella and Jelly

Peanut butter is a common staple in many homes; my own daughter eats a peanut butter and jelly sandwich every day for lunch. As I spread the creamy goodness on the bread, the last thing that I want to think about is that I may be spreading *Salmonella* as well. After all, this pathogen has been linked to poultry, eggs, and dirty water, how could it possibly get into commercially sealed peanut butter?

This was just the question that the CDC was asking in November 2006 when they noted an unusual increase in foodborne illness linked to *Salmonella* Tennessee. This is one of the rarer serotypes of the pathogen, so it was relatively easy for the CDC to trace the source of the illnesses back to one common source: peanut butter. Over a nine-month period, starting in August 2006, the CDC confirmed 628 cases of illness in 47 states associated with *Salmonella* Tennessee.[27]

How did *Salmonella* get into jars of peanut butter? Environmental health professionals are still trying to answer this question. After the outbreak investigation was complete, it was clear that the affected peanut butter was packaged in only one plant—ConAgra's Sylvester, Georgia plant. The peanut butter involved was sold under both Peter Pan and Great Value brand names. According to the FDA, the Peter Pan brand was distributed to more than 60 countries, while the Great Value brand was only distributed in the United States at Wal-Mart stores.

According to the CDC, this was the first time that peanut butter was implicated as the mode of transmission for a foodborne pathogen in the United States. In addition, the Tennessee serotype of *Salmonella* is rarely found to be a contributor to widespread illness. Although the CDC has not definitively answered the question of how the peanut butter became contaminated, there are several probable scenarios. First, bacteria could have found their way into the raw peanuts at any point in the growing cycle. This can occur if the peanuts are irrigated with dirty water or if animals come in close contact with the peanuts. The CDC has ruled this scenario out in this case because only one processing plant was involved, and the peanuts used at this plant were used at other plants without any documented problems.

Ruling out raw peanuts as the source suggests that conditions at the processing facility created the opportunity for bacteria to get into the peanut butter. It is likely that at some point in the production process, *Salmonella* was introduced into peanut butter. This could have occurred as the peanuts were being stored prior to processing if rodents or other animals defecated on them. Even if rodents in the plant did contaminate the peanuts, the peanuts are heated and roasted before they are ground into peanut butter, a process that would normally kill bacterial pathogens. However, *Salmonella* can survive high temperatures and prefers high-fat foods, so peanut butter is actually an excellent medium for the growth of these bacteria. If rodents in the plant were not the source of the *Salmonella*, then the only other plausible scenario has the peanut butter becoming tainted while it was being made.

If the theory that the bacteria got into the jars during the processing is true, it may be that the jars themselves were not sterile. Recall that these bacteria are spread by feces, so the source of the bacteria could have been inadequately treated water used throughout the peanut butter processing. The other logical source of the pathogen is a sick person who worked in the processing facility. Environmental health professionals will continue to investigate how the peanut butter was contaminated, but it is likely that the exact cause of the outbreak will never be known.

Even though the 2006 outbreak was the first in the United States to be associated with peanut butter, *Salmonella* had been linked to peanut butter in other countries prior to this event. For example, in 1996 there was an outbreak of salmonellosis linked to peanut butter in Australia.[28] The Australian outbreak prompted researchers to explore the viability of these bacteria in peanut butter. After infecting peanut butter that they purchased in retail stores and monitoring levels of *Salmonella* over time, they concluded that once these bacteria find their way into peanut butter, they are likely to remain viable for long periods of time.

Although the first case of *Salmonella* food poisoning in the U.S. outbreak was identified in August 2006, it wasn't until February 2007 that the CDC was able to make the link between peanut butter and sick people. It was at this time, in February 2007, that the manufacturer, ConAgra, issued its recall, almost six months after the outbreak started. Remember that recalls are voluntary, not mandatory, and the FDA does not have the authority to require a company to recall a product that may be a public health threat. It is logical that a manufacturer would be cautious about issuing a recall notice because to some this may seem like an admission that the company is accepting responsibility for the situation. This perception of responsibility, and the search for a culpably party, leads to lawsuits and bad publicity, both outcomes that could affect the bottom line of the industry involved.

In addition to possibly opening the door to litigation, a recall can be expensive. ConAgra understands the seriousness of being involved in a recall as it pertains to their bottom line. Their 2007 annual report says this about the peanut butter recall, "during the third quarter of fiscal 2007, the Company initiated a voluntary recall of all varieties of peanut butter manufactured at its Sylvester, Georgia plant. The costs of the recall negatively impacted net sales, gross margin, and operating profit in the Consumer Foods and International Foods segments in fiscal 2007, and the Company expects ongoing impacts to its business in early fiscal 2008. A number of lawsuits and claims related to the recalled product have been filed against the Company."[29]

The lawsuits mentioned in the annual report related to the peanut butter outbreak and subsequent recall are being led by several law firms who advertise their services to those who were made ill by eating the product. The creation of the Web site "peanutbutter-lawsuitlawyer.com" is one example of a law firm that is offering free consultations to anyone who got sick from eating peanut butter. There is also "peanutbutterclassaction.com," created by a law firm that filed a class action lawsuit against ConAgra three days after the voluntary recall. The fact that recalls are voluntary and litigation is often swift after a recall leads to speculation that the recalls that are actually implemented may be indicative of only a small fraction of the actual problems with food processing.

Is ConAgra just unlucky when it comes to food safety? Is the company involved in unsafe food processing practices? Or, is someone out to get this company by intentionally contaminating some of its most popular products? These questions have to be raised because just as the peanut butter outbreak was winding down, a new problem emerged from a different ConAgra food processing facility, involving a completely difference food and strain of *Salmonella*.

A *Salmonella* Banquet

One Banquet chicken pot pie has 380 calories, and 21 grams of fat, eight of which are saturated fat, constituting about 41 percent of your recommended daily intake of saturated fat. In addition, there are 841 milligrams of sodium in one pot pie, which is about 35 percent of your recommended intake. In 2007, some pot pies contained more than your recommended daily intake of *Salmonella* too. ConAgra was again implicated as the source of diarrhea in almost 300 people who had eaten pot pies.

ConAgra foods is a huge corporation encompassing brands such as Banquet, Chef Boyardee, Healthy Choice, Libby's, Pam, and Wesson. According to its 2007 Annual Report, which is available on its Web site, the company posted more than $12 billion in sales from May 2006 to May 2007, for a net profit of more than $3 billion. ConAgra's headquarters are in Omaha, Nebraska, and it has more than 200 manufacturing facilities across the country. The peanut butter outbreak originated in its plant in Sylvester, Georgia, but the pot pie outbreak was linked to its plant in Marshall, Missouri.

In the pot pie outbreak, the CDC identified the strain as *Salmonella* I 4,[5],12:i:-.[30] This strain is also known as *Salmonella enterica* subspecies *enterica* Serotype 4,5,12:i:- (recall that group I *Salmonella* is the *enterica* subspecies). This serotype is a variant of *Salmonella* Typhimurium and is relatively rare. It is not common in foodborne outbreaks, and recent outbreaks have included cases that occurred as a result of exposure to live poultry. For example, this strain was identified as the cause of illness in an outbreak from exposure to baby chicks at an agricultural feed store in Michigan in 2006 in which 21 people were reported ill and seven of the victims required hospitalization.[31] Some of the sick people were children who had just picked up baby chicks; others had taken some chicks home and were made sick then.

Salmonella I 4,[5],12:i:- is a relatively new strain. However, there has been a notable increase in cases of gastrointestinal illness in which this pathogen has been identified as the cause of the illness since the late 1990s in both the United States and in Spain. Spain identified this strain in 1997 and noted its ability to resist multiple antibiotics used to treat *Salmonella* infections.[32] The first documented U.S. outbreak of illness linked to this strain occurred in New York City in 1998.[33]

ConAgra issued a recall notice in October 2007 for pot pies produced under a variety of brand names including several grocery story brands such as Kroger and Meijer. Pot pies were recalled in at least 30 states, amounting to about $30 million worth of product. The investigation as to how this strain of *Salmonella* made it into pot pies is ongoing as of the writing of this book. However, it is conceivable that the meat in the pot pies was the source of the pathogen. Remember that poultry is a common carrier of *Salmonella* and it is likely that the pot pies were not processed in a manner adequate to destroy the pathogen. What is interesting about this outbreak is that the bacteria were able to survive the freezing process.

If the pathogen was not killed during processing and the pot pies were allowed to thaw anytime during their trip to the grocery stores, the bacteria could have easily reproduced. However, because of the involvement of so many states with this outbreak, it is not likely that transportation errors played a significant role in the incidence of contaminated pot pies. If it had, the implication would be that numerous trucks were deficient in their ability to maintain safe temperatures, not a real probable scenario.

Once the pot pies arrived at the groceries, it was up to the grocer to ensure that they remained frozen, or optimal conditions for pathogen growth could ensue. If the product is not kept frozen, then the bacteria could begin their exponential reproduction. Again because of the magnitude of this outbreak, it is unlikely that groceries in all of the states involved were incompetent in receiving and storing frozen food. So if it wasn't the manufacturer, the transporter, or the grocer who contributed to levels of *Salmonella* that were high enough to make people sick, then who was it?

Ultimately, ConAgra suggested that a major contributing factor to the disease outbreak was that the consumers of these pot pies must not have cooked them correctly. Most bacteria will be killed during cooking, and microwaving a pot pie according to package directions should create high enough temperatures to kill *Salmonella*. In their press release about the recall, ConAgra reminded consumers that the pot pies were not a "ready-to-eat" food and that they must be cooked thoroughly to ensure their safety.

The most reasonable scenario in the pot pie outbreak is that the pot pies were contaminated at the processing plant and that consumers did not cook them to high enough temperatures to ensure that the pathogens were killed. In November the facility where the pot pies were produced began making them again, after being closed for several weeks. The USDA official who was responsible for inspecting the plant said that ConAgra had made improvements in two areas that may have contributed to the contamination.

On November 27, 2007, Dean Hollis, the ConAgra executive who was responsible for the division that manufactures its peanut butter and pot pies, resigned. He had been employed at ConAgra since 1987 and took over control of the Consumer Foods Group Division in 2005. ConAgra also updated their instructions for cooking pot pies and now cautions consumers to cook the pies in accordance with the wattage of their microwave ovens and to use a meat thermometer to test the internal temperature of the pot pie. These new instructions suggest that everybody knows the wattage of their microwave and that there is a working, calibrated food thermometer in every kitchen. The new instructions will probably not offer much additional protection to consumers, but they should help protect the company from further lawsuits.

Scrambled *Salmonella*

Peanut butter and pot pies are not usually foods associated with *Salmonella*; eggs are. Remember the scene in the movie *Rocky* when Sylvester

Stallone's character drinks a glass of raw eggs? At the time I first saw the movie, I thought it was gross; now, I think it was probably deadly. Raw eggs have been a known source of *Salmonella* for a long time. The strain of the bacteria that is most common in eggs is *Salmonella* Enteritidis (i.e., *Salmonella enterica* serovar Enteritidis) or SE.

Raw eggs are components of salad dressings and many sauces, such as Caesar salad dressing and hollandaise sauce, because of their ability to both bind and thicken. Finding products with raw eggs as a component is becoming increasingly rare due to governmental guidance. The FDA recommends never eating undercooked or runny eggs, basing this recommendation on research that identified SE in the yolks of eggs. Studies show that SE can get into the yolk before the shell is formed, in addition to being deposited in the shell as the egg is laid.[34]

The FDA warning has now been translated onto restaurant menus across the country. If you read your menu carefully the next time you eat out, pay attention to phrases that warn you about eating undercooked eggs or sauces that contain these eggs. Presumably these phrases are on menus to limit the liability of any food service establishment if someone should get sick, since the warnings do nothing to actually improve the safety of eggs.

FROM DIARRHEA TO ARTHRITIS

In addition to acute health effects such as diarrhea, *Salmonella* has been associated with at least two chronic health conditions, the first being Guillain-Barré syndrome (GBS).[35] GBS is a rare disease that manifests itself in the form of muscle weakness and is also associated with eating foods contaminated with *Campylobacter*, a pathogen that is discussed in Chapter 6. There appears to be a link between at least one infectious agent and this disease, and *Salmonella* is a likely suspect because of its known association with arthritis.

Arthritis is one chronic disease that has been connected to *Salmonella* poisoning. Specifically, it is accepted by the scientific community that rheumatoid arthritis is caused by bacterial infections.[36] In addition, there are numerous case studies that implicate *Salmonella* in worsening the conditions of arthritis sufferers. In one case, a patient who had a severe form of arthritis and was in remission suffered a setback two weeks after having been infected with one strain of *Salmonella*.[37] Although other bacterial pathogens that cause gastroenteritis are known to be associated with arthritis, *Salmonella* is the one that has been most often found in patients who are suffering from arthritis after an enteric illness.[38]

LEADING DOWN THE PATH TO ANTIBIOTIC RESISTANCE

There is evidence that antibiotic use in animals to prevent contamination of our food supply is higher than human use to treat illness.[39] This is especially the case in poultry farming. Studies have shown that bacteria are prevalent in chickens slaughtered for the food supply, and many of the species of *Salmonella* identified in market poultry are resistant to common antibiotics.[40] Antibiotic resistance in foods contaminated with *Salmonella* is extremely threatening to public health since these bacteria continue to be among the leading causes of foodborne illness worldwide. If we ingest antibiotic-resistant strains of this pathogen and get sick, we may not respond to antibiotics to treat the illness. In addition, our consumption of antibiotic-resistant bacteria is contributing to a larger, global threat of antibiotic resistance.

Wisconsin is known as "America's Dairyland" because of its abundance of dairy farms. It is also a hotbed of *Salmonella* Newport activity, a strain related to consumption of unpasteurized dairy products. As such, the state offers opportunities to study ongoing cases of *Salmonella*, and one such study was conducted on cases of *Salmonella* Newport reported from 2003 to 2005. The researchers were looking for signs of antibiotic resistance in this strain, and they found it. The numbers of multidrug-resistant cases of *Salmonella* Newport were significantly higher in Wisconsin than in the rest of the country as a whole. The high levels of resistance discovered led the researchers to suggest that greater efforts need to be made to monitor antibiotic resistance of *Salmonella* in states that are major producers of our dairy supply.[41]

Meanwhile, across the country in the state of Washington, researchers have identified a potential problem with a strain of *Salmonella enterica* serovar Typhimurium.[42] In their comparison of bovine and human cases of this strain, they have identified a new multidrug-resistant clone that is currently contained to the Pacific Northwest. However, based on historical trends with *Salmonella* species, it is possible that this strain could migrate to other parts of the country, threatening public health. As if peanut butter and pot pies were not enough, additional nationwide outbreaks of *Salmonella* occurred in 2006 and 2007, and pet food, snack food, and tomatoes were the source of the bacteria.

Combined with the problem of antibiotic resistance is the emergence of outbreaks associated with rare strains of *Salmonella*. In August 2007, dry pet food was the source of one outbreak of *Salmonella* serotype Schwarzengrund. More than 60 people in multiple states were confirmed infected with this strain of the bacteria, and the investigation revealed that people who were sick had purchased the same type of dry pet food. *Salmonella* serotype Wandsworth, which is another rare form of the bacteria, caused illness in more than 65 people in 20 states in the summer of 2007. A snack food called "Veggie Booty" was the food implicated as the cause of this outbreak. In the fall of 2006 more than 180 people in several states were confirmed sick with *Salmonella* Typhimurium. These people had been exposed to the bacteria by eating tomatoes at restaurants.

SEARCHING FOR *SALMONELLA*

One of the best ways to address the increasing burden of *Salmonella* food poisoning is by enhanced surveillance. If public health professionals are able to identify and investigate outbreaks quickly and efficiently, the number of cases of illness could be minimized. The WHO began a program in the year 2000 to strengthen the ability of the global public health system to respond to foodborne illness and to specifically identify emerging strains of *Salmonella* that are antibiotic resistant.

Global Salm Surv (GSS) is a partnership among several countries to quickly disseminate scientific information about strains of *Salmonella* that are involved in foodborne outbreaks.[43] The goals of GSS include conducting international training on laboratory techniques for identifying types of the pathogen, developing guidance on laboratory quality assurance, establishing regional centers that would offer training and research relevant to regional conditions, and providing a forum for discussion and information exchange among public health professionals across the globe. As of 2006, there were 138 countries represented in GSS and four regional centers.

As with many programs developed to prevent disease, especially those that focus on surveillance such as GSS, resources are the critical factor in ensuring success. In the fall of 2005, members of GSS met in Canada to review the accomplishments of their first five years and to plan for the next five.[44] From 2000 to 2005 GSS was successful in conducting international training and providing quality assurance at numerous laboratories. In addition, GSS identified three strains of *Salmonella* as the most common cause of *Salmonella*-related illness reported in the network: Enteriditis, Typhimurium, and Newport.

As for the future of GSS, the discussion at the meeting centered on the need to ensure adequate funding to accomplish the goals for 2006–2010. Most of the countries expressed concern over their ability to continue meaningful participation in the face of competing demands for their public health resources. Although the meeting did result in new goals for GSS, it is uncertain whether these goals will be achieved due to resource constraints.

NOTES

1. J. Michael Janda and Sharon L. Abbott, *The Enterobacteria,* 2nd ed. (Washington, DC: ASM Press, 2005).

2. Calvin M. Kunin, "Urinary-Catheter-Associated Infections in the Elderly," *International Journal of Antimicrobial Agents* 28S (2006): S78–S81.

3. B. J. Tindall et al., "Nomenclature and Taxonomy of the Genus *Salmonella,*" *International Journal of Systemic and Evolutionary Microbiology* 55 (2005): 521–24.

4. R. E. Buchanan, Ralph St. John-Brooks, and Robert S. Breed, eds., "International Bacteriological Code of Nomenclature," *Journal of Bacteriology* 55, no. 3 (1948): 287–306.

5. CDC, *Salmonella Surveillance: Annual Summary 2005,* http://www.cdc.gov/ncidod/dbmd/phlisdata/salmonella.htm.

6. Mark Heyndrickx, et al., "Recent Changes in *Salmonella* Nomenclature: The Need for Clarification," *The Veterinary Journal* 170 (2005): 275–77.

7. CDC, *Salmonella Surveillance: Annual Summary 2005.*

8. This bureau became the Agricultural Research Service in 1953.

9. National Archives, *Records of the Bureau of Animal Industry,* http://www.archives.gov/research/guide-fed-records/groups/017.html#17.

10. Whonamedit.com, "Daniel Salmon," http://www.whonamedit.com/doctor.cfm/408.html (accessed January 21, 2008).

11. Claude E. Doman and Richard J. Wolfe, *Suppressing the Diseases of Animals and Man: Theobald Smith, Microbiologist* (Boston: Harvard University Press, 2003).

12. George Hormis Lorimer, "Servant of Mankind," *Saturday Evening Post* 207, no. 37 (1935): 26.

13. Manolis J. Papagrigorakis, et al., "Ancient Typhoid Epidemic Reveals Possible Ancestral Strain of *Salmonella enterica* serovar Typhi," *Infection, Genetics and Evolution* 7 (2007): 126–27; Manolis J. Papagrigorakis, et al., "DNA Examination of Ancient Dental Pulp Incriminates Typhoid Fever as Probable Cause of the Plague of Athens," *International Journal of Infectious Diseases* 10 (2006): 206–14.

14. The History Guide, "Thucydides on the Athenian Plague of 430 B.C.," http://www.historyguide.org/ancient/athenian_plague.html (accessed January 21, 2008).

15. Medline Plus Medical Encyclopedia, "Typhoid Fever," http://www.nlm.nih.gov/medlineplus/ency/article/001332.htm (accessed January 21, 2008).

16. Beth Shapiro, Andrew Rambaut, and M. Thomas P. Gilbert, "No Proof that Typhoid Causes the Plague of Athens (A Reply to Papagrigorakis et al.), *International Journal of Infectious Diseases* 10 (2006): 334–40.

17. Victor M. Parachin, "Typhoid Mary: 'The Most Dangerous Woman in America'," *American History* 40 (2006): 24–26.

18. See for example, "The Work of a Chronic Typhoid Germ Distributor, George A. Soper, Ph.D.," http://www.learner.org/channel/workshops/primarysources/disease/docs/soper.html; and "The Most Dangerous Woman in America," http://www.pbs.org/wgbh/nova/typhoid/.

19. E. B. Steinberg et al., "Typhoid Fever in Travelers: Who Should Be Targeted for Prevention?" *Clinical Infectious Diseases* 39 (2004):186–91.

20. Buddha Basnyat et al., "Enteric (Typhoid) Fever in Travelers," *Clinical Infectious Diseases* 41 (2005): 1467–72.

21. CDC, *Traveler's Health Yellow Book,* http://wwwn.cdc.gov/travel/yellowBookCh4-Typhoid.aspx.

22. World Health Organization, "Typhoid Fever," http://www.who.int/topics/typhoid_fever/en/.

23. Abigail Fraser et al., "Typhoid Fever Vaccines: Systematic Review and Meta-Analysis of Randomised Controlled Trials," *Vaccine* 25 (2007): 7848–57.

24. Volga Punda-Polić, "War-Associated Cases of Typhoid Fever Imported to Split-Dalmatia County (Croatia), *Military Medicine* 172, no. 10 (2007): 1096–98.

25. Elisabeth R. Benjamin et al., "The Humanitarian Cost of War," *The Lancet* 361, no. 9360 (2003): 874; Paroma Basu, "Iraq's Public Health Infrastructure a Casualty of War," *Nature Medicine* 10, no. 2 (2004): 110.

26. Philippe Roumagnac et al., "Evolutionary History of *Salmonella* Typhi," *Science* 314: 1301–4.

27. CDC, "Multistate Outbreak of *Salmonella* Tennessee Infections Associated with Peanut Butter—United States, 2006–2007," *Morbidity and Mortality Weekly Report* 56, no. 21 (2007): 521–24.

28. S. L. Burnett et al., "Survival of *Salmonella* in Peanut Butter and Peanut Butter Spread," *Journal of Applied Microbiology* 89 (2000): 472–77.

29. ConAgra Foods Inc., 2007 Annual Report, http://thomson.mobular.net/thomson/7/2480/2791/.

30. This may look unusual, but the way this strain is written is: 4,5,12:i:-.

31. CDC, "Three Outbreaks of Salmonellosis Associated with Baby Poultry from Three Hatcheries—United States, 2006," *Morbidity and Mortality Weekly Report* 56, no. 12 (2007): 273–76.

32. María Luisa Güerri et al., "Detection of Integrons and Antibiotic-Resistance Genes in *Salmonella enterica* serovar Typhimurium Isolates with Resistance to Ampicillin and Variable Susceptibility to Amoxicillin-Clavulanate," *International Journal of Antimicrobial Agents* 24 (2004): 327–33.

33. Alice Agasan et al., "Profile of *Salmonella enterica* subsp. *enterica* (subspecies I) serotype 4, 5, 12:i:- Strains Causing Foodborne Infection in New York City," *Journal of Clinical Microbiology* 40 (2002): 1924–29.

34. K. De Reu et al., "Eggshell Factors Influencing Eggshell Penetration and Whole Egg Contamination by Different Bacteria Including *Salmonella enteritidis*," *International Journal of Food Microbiology* 112 (2006): 253–60.

35. Fahmi Yousef Khan et al., "Guillain-Barré Syndrome Associated with *Salmonella paratyphi*." *Clinical Neurology and Neurosurgery* 109 (2007): 452–54.

36. J. D. Carter and L. R. Espinoza, "Interplay of Environmental Triggers and Host Response in Reactive Arthritis: Can We Intervene?" *Future Rheumatology* 1 (2006): 717–27.

37. L. Punzi et al., "Psoriatic Arthritis Exacerbated by *Salmonella* Infection," *Clinical Rheumatology* 19 (2000): 167–68.

38. J. S. Hill Gaston and M. S. Lillicrap, "Arthritis Associated with Enteric Infection," *Best Practice & Research. Clinical Rheumatology* 17 (2003): 219–39.

39. Herbert L. DuPont, "The Growing Threat of Foodborne Bacterial Enteropathogens of Animal Origin," *Clinical Infectious Diseases* 45 (2007): 1353–61.

40. R. Capita, C. Alonso-Calleja, and M. Prieto, "Prevalence of *Salmonella enterica* Serovars and Genovars from Chicken Carcasses in Slaughterhouses in Spain," *Journal of Applied Microbiology* 103 (2007): 1366–75; D. J. Bolton et al., "A Survey for Serotyping, Antibiotic Resistance Profiling and PFGE Characterization of and the Potential Multiplication of Restaurant *Salmonella* Isolates," *Journal of Applied Microbiology* 103 (2007): 1681–90; Thi Thu Hao Van et al., "Detection of *Salmonella* spp. in Retail Raw Food Samples from Vietnam and Characterization of Their Antibiotic Resistance," *Applied and Environmental Microbiology* 73 (2007): 6885–90.

41. Amy E. Karon et al., "Human Multi-Drug Resistant *Salmonella* Newport Infections, Wisconsin, 2003–2005," *Emerging Infectious Diseases* (2007), http://www.cdc.gov/eid/content/13/11/1777.htm.

42. Margaret A. Davis et al., "Multidrug-Resistant *Salmonella* Typhimurium, Pacific Northwest, United States," *Emerging Infectious Diseases* (2007), http://www.cdc.gov/eid/content/13/10/contents_v13n10.htm.

43. World Health Organization, *Global Salm Surv,* http://www.who.int/salmsurv/en/ (accessed January 9, 2008).

44. World Health Organization, *WHO Global Salm-Surv Strategic Plan 2006–2010* (Geneva, Switzerland: WHO, 2006), http://www.who.int/salmsurv/general/documents/GSS_STRATEGICPLAN2006_10.pdf.

— 4 —

Floating Viruses

Anyone who is a parent knows the feeling when your child wakes you to tell you that she/he has a stomachache. Sometimes you wait it out, with hopes that it will go away on its own. But when the stomachache turns into diarrhea, some parents may become alarmed enough to call their doctor. Many parents probably won't send their kids to school. So imagine the situation on an October day in 1968 in a small community in northeast Ohio when more than one hundred elementary school children told their parents they weren't feeling well. Most of the children started vomiting and had watery diarrhea, which in some cases may have lasted for as long as five days. Officials in the school district knew there was a problem because there were only about two hundred students enrolled in the elementary school and almost half of them reported that they would be absent in a period of a couple of days.

Health officials and researchers also realized that they were involved in a major outbreak of a common illness, so they saved samples of stool from some of the kids who had visited their doctors. The samples were sent to labs at the CDC and researchers began to analyze the samples almost immediately. However, it wasn't until 1972 that microbiologists identified a new pathogen in the samples, and this one was not a bacterium, it was a virus. Ultimately, this outbreak led to one of the most important discoveries in the study of foodborne illness, because the virus that was identified in 1972 is now known to be the leading cause of nonbacterial diarrhea. The small town in northeast Ohio will never be forgotten because, as is the case with many microbiological discoveries, this virus was named after the place it was first identified and was labeled "Norwalk Virus," after Norwalk, Ohio.

The discovery in 1972 of a viral cause of gastrointestinal illness was especially significant because viruses are much more difficult to identify than bacteria for at least three reasons: (1) they do not grow on cultures in a lab like bacteria; (2) they do not reproduce in foods, so they are not as easy to spot as bacteria; and (3) many labs that test food samples for microbiological pathogens do not routinely test for viruses.[1] The microbiological study of viruses is called "virology" and, although the science emerged in the late nineteenth century, there is evidence that viruses have been the cause of disease for thousands of years.

A BRIEF HISTORY OF VIRUSES

In discussions of the history of virology, it is common to find a picture of an Egyptian hieroglyph.[2] There appears to be some disagreement about who the picture depicts and the timing of the hieroglyph, but it appears most likely that it depicts Temple Priest Ruma and is from about 3000 B.C. The hieroglyph shows a grown man using a crutch because of a deformity that makes his right leg shorter than his left, a symptom that we now know a consequence of polio. Further evidence of the long history of polio was found in 1905 when the tomb of the Egyptian King Siptah, who ruled from 1193 to 1187 B.C., was discovered.

When Siptah's remains were found, one leg was clearly shorter than the other. Historical records indicate that Siptah was not born with the deformity that made his right leg shorter than his left, leading to the theory that his problem was caused by some type of disease. The deformity could have been the result of infection with the polio virus. From these historical findings and other similar accounts, scientists have deduced that viruses have probably been a significant cause of illness for thousands of years.

Even though there is some indication that polio could have been responsible for human suffering in ancient Egypt, the first clinical description of the disease was not published until 1789 when a British physician, Michael Underwood, described deformities in children.[3] At the time Underwood wrote his account of the symptoms, there were no clear data to suggest that an infectious virus was the cause of the irregularities in the children. There was ongoing research related to polio and smallpox in the late 1700s, but it wasn't until 1898 that a nonbacterial agent of disease was actually identified.

Two German scientists, Freidrich Loeffler and Paul Frosch, reported that they had identified the cause of foot-and-mouth disease in cattle and that the organism was not a bacterium.[4] They reported that the pathogen was much smaller than bacteria, but that they were able to capture it and demonstrate its ability to transmit the disease among animals. This discovery was one of the most important in the realm of virology, ultimately leading to the labeling of Loeffler and Frosch as the "founders of animal virology."[5]

Virology as a science is a critical component of understanding infectious diseases, especially considering that viruses cause a large percentage of global illness including influenza, HIV/AIDS, hepatitis, and encephalitis. Viruses can be classified using several characteristics including their structure, the types of cells they infect, and their genetic makeup. There are 25 known families of viruses and at least 60 different genera. Viruses are smaller than bacteria, a fact that makes them more difficult to identify with basic microbiological techniques. Many viruses cannot be seen without the aid of an electron microscope, and in some instances it is only possible to identify the virus by using techniques to isolate their genetic material.

Viruses are made up of DNA and RNA surrounded by a shell of protein. In order for viruses to survive they must find a living host that is carrying susceptible cells. Once in the host, the virus gets inside susceptible cells and uses these cells to replicate. Many viruses have specific tastes in that they will invade only the cells that will be the most beneficial to their survival. For example, the virus that causes hepatitis only goes after cells in the liver. Often the result of the viral invasion is that the cell dies and symptoms occur in the host as the normal cells are replaced with viruses.

Because viruses cannot survive unless they find cells in which to replicate, they are always on the lookout for willing hosts. In terms of human viral infection, some viruses can wait for extended periods of time on computer keyboards, on telephone receivers, in food and water, and even in the air until a host ingests or inhales them. Once inside the body, the virus may take its time looking for the right cells and most opportune moment to begin its attack. This is the reason why there can be some very long delays from the time a person is exposed to the time symptoms develop. It is possible to be infected with viruses, but to not have symptoms of the disease that they cause; that is, to just be carriers of viruses. People aid virus survival by not washing their hands frequently enough, by eating food that has not been cooked thoroughly, and by drinking unsafe water. When it comes to most viral diseases in humans, we have been accomplices in their spread and evolution.

THE TRIP FROM NORWALK, OHIO

Almost 40 years after the discovery of the virus in northeastern Ohio, the Norwalk virus has been implicated in sickening hundreds of thousands of people across the globe. The Norwalk virus is now classified into a group called noroviruses. Noroviruses are considered to be the leading cause of nonbacterial diarrhea and there are almost daily accounts of norovirus outbreaks. In 2007, it was possible to identify at least one outbreak of norovirus per month in the United States alone, including the following:[6]

- January: A Hilton hotel outside of Washington, D.C, was forced to close for several days after several hotel guests became ill. The Health Department identified a food service worker as the likely source of the virus.
- February: Norovirus was confirmed as the cause of illness in at least 35 people in St. Petersburg, Florida. The ill people had either eaten lunch at a local café or food catered by the café at a county commissioner's event.
- March: More than 300 patients and staff at the Hebrew Rehabilitation Center near Boston were diagnosed with acute gastrointestinal illness that was identified as a norovirus. About 28 percent of the patient population was sick and at least one death was thought to be caused by the virus.
- April: Thirty percent of the students at Augusta Middle School in Butler County, Kansas, stayed home from school on one day in April. The local health department conducted an investigation and implicated norovirus spread through contaminated cafeteria food.
- May: About 20 people at a nursing home in Washington, North Carolina, were sickened and the likely cause was norovirus.
- June: At least 60 people called the Cowitz County Health Department reporting symptoms indicative of norovirus after eating at a local restaurant in Longview, Washington.
- July: More than 60 people got ill after swimming in a pool at West Chester University near Philadelphia. Tests of the pool water confirmed fecal contamination of the water and the presence of norovirus.
- August: The Oregon State Hospital reports that about 170 people, patients and staff, had symptoms of norovirus.
- September: As many as 50 people suffered from exposure to norovirus after staying in a Holiday Inn hotel near Harrisburg, Pennsylvania.
- October: An elementary school in Eaton Rapids, Michigan, reported that almost 25 percent of the students were out sick in one day.
- November: An outbreak in Redwood Falls, Minnesota, sickened at least 54 people and was linked to a Burger King restaurant.
- December: An outbreak in East Lyme, Connecticut led to the closing of all public schools on December 20, 2007.

The noroviruses are now considered a leading cause of acute gastroenteritis (AGE)—that is, diarrhea—in the United States, and perhaps most of the developed countries across the globe. Many environmental health professionals believe that of all of the foodborne pathogens, noroviruses are the most important. They are easily spread and can stay in the environment for long periods of time. It is possible to pick up these viruses from food, inanimate objects, or directly from a person who is ill. Regardless of how norovirus is contracted, the reason for the spread is simple: people do not wash their hands well, or at all, after using the bathroom.

Norovirus is similar to *Salmonella* in that it is known as a "fecal" pathogen. However, unlike *Salmonella*, it is found in human feces rather than animal feces. This means that if it is in your food, it got there from somebody's feces rather than from poor slaughterhouse techniques or contaminated eggs. The only way this is likely to happen is if the carrier does not practice good hygiene. One person who does not wash his or her hands after using the bathroom can sicken hundreds of people, especially if this person is a food service worker. Outbreaks are often associated with facilities that employ hourly, low-wage workers, such as fast-food restaurants, nursing homes, and schools. Often these food service workers continue to work even if they are sick because they do not have paid sick leave and they need the money.

The Leading Cause of "Stomach Flu"

In surveying environmental health professionals across the country, I found that most of the stories that they want to share about outbreaks are related to norovirus. Since many environmental health professionals believe that noroviruses are the most important cause of foodborne disease outbreaks in the country, they are quick to share stories of some of the outbreaks that they have been involved with that have ultimately been linked to norovirus. For example, one environmental health professional told the story of a bartender who vomited at work, but tended bar at a Christmas party because he thought the tips would be good. The result was that many partygoers got sick even though the bartender did not handle food, he only served drinks.[7]

Another environmental health professional explained the case of one food service employee who had been out of town at a family reunion and came into work to tell his managers that he had the "stomach flu" and couldn't work. While waiting in the kitchen to speak to the manager, he vomited in a garbage can. He did not shake any hands, prepare any food, or touch anything other than the garbage bag he threw up in (which he promptly took outside to the dumpster). Patrons of the restaurant who ate ready-to-eat foods from the salad preparation area near the garbage can where he threw up became ill. In addition, several of his coworkers who were working at the facility the day he was in developed similar symptoms. Since none of the foods served to the sick customers and employees were prepared or even touched by the one sick employee, this situation illustrates a possible example of how this virus can be spread through the air.

There was also the case of one member of the kitchen staff in an assisted living facility who had diarrhea and was vomiting one day. She returned to work the next day because most of the kitchen staff was sick and she felt she would be needed. Her concern over making sure that the meals for the residents of the facility were taken care of led to the spread of diarrheal illness rapidly through the facility.

Then there was the ill woman who cut bread for a school dinner that would serve about 200 children. She knew she was sick so she decided to help out by only cutting bread for the meal, thinking it would not be a problem to work with the bread because it is not a "usual suspect" on the list of foods that normally spread germs. When she was finished cutting the bread, she went home because she was feeling worse. The next morning at least 158 children were ill and the school was shut down for a period of time to allow the kids to recover. Closing schools on account of the norovirus is becoming an increasingly common event, and it is not just primary and secondary schools that are affected.

The Virus Goes to School

Norovirus often strikes in schools, assisted living centers, and other institutional settings. Living and working conditions in most institutions create an environment that is highly conducive to the spread of numerous infectious agents. There are many people in close quarters and, when it comes to children especially, sanitation and hygiene are sometimes not a personal priority. In general, viruses will be easy to spread in these settings because of their ability to survive for extended periods of time on inanimate objects.

In 2007, there were numerous outbreaks of norovirus that led to school closures including one in May that closed a middle school in Kalamazoo, Michigan, for three days. An outbreak in September shut down schools in a suburb of Chicago. The virus took down almost the entire high school football team in Jefferson County, Colorado, in November. Also in November, an elementary school in Chester, Connecticut, was closed after more than half of the students were absent with symptoms of norovirus. When the virus is prevalent enough to close schools, we hear about it in the media, but what about when the virus affects other learning institutions, such as colleges?

Responding to an online survey, one environmental health professional working for a local health department explained that an investigation of an outbreak at one university began when a food service manager in a large dorm called the health department at 8 A.M. one Wednesday morning in a panic. He said, "Please come over and help me. I've had phone calls from 26 students saying they were vomiting all last night and I don't know what to do." The cases were clustered in certain living areas, so it was evident most of the victims were friends with each other. The following Monday, an outbreak of similar symptoms among members of a student club that had met the previous Friday emerged—two days after the dorm outbreak. Only cookies and lemonade had been served at the meeting, so there was no chance that the illness was caused by undercooked meat or other hazardous foods. The environmental health investigation uncovered that the student who had mixed and poured lemonade and arranged cookies with his bare hands had been ill two days earlier in the previous dorm outbreak.

If you are sick with diarrhea and perhaps vomiting, it is highly likely that the cause of your illness is a norovirus. This is so often the cause of acute diarrhea that it has become known as the "stomach virus"; we also refer to it as the "stomach flu." Remember that viruses are different from bacteria in terms of their ability to reproduce. That is, it is often not possible to use the principles of time and temperature control to minimize the spread of viruses in food. This is clearly demonstrated when viruses are spread by people who touch ready-to-eat foods that will not be cooked further. Some of the more interesting outbreaks of norovirus have occurred in fast-food restaurants, in recreational fountains that children play in, and during major natural disasters.

SUBMARINE SANDWICHES, RECREATIONAL FOUNTAINS, AND DISASTERS

When two or more people are ill from eating a common food, environmental public health officials call the sickness an outbreak. There were 372 outbreaks of AGE reported to the CDC between October and December 2005.[8] Between October and December 2006, 1,316 outbreaks were reported, a 254 percent increase from the previous year. Of the 1,316 outbreaks in 2006, 382 or 29 percent were confirmed to be caused by norovirus. Many of the remaining 71 percent of the outbreaks could not identify a common cause. In some of the norovirus outbreaks a single food handler was implicated; in others the source of the pathogen was environmental.

One outbreak involved a national submarine sandwich chain in Michigan and was caused by an ill food handler.[9] The reason the food handler worked while sick is because the small restaurant couldn't spare the employee during a busy period. This scenario is often compounded by the fact that employees in many of these types of restaurants do not have paid sick time, so there are no incentives for them to take a day off when ill. In this situation, one sick food handler infected people attending at least three different events. One of these was among people who had attended a school activity, the second involved staff at a publishing company, and the third included members of a civic organization. All three groups ate party-sized sandwiches, and numerous people in all three groups became ill. At the school luncheon, 23 of the 29 staff who attended the meal got sick. This case provides evidence of how one person can threaten public health.

Public health can also be threatened by norovirus in ways that are the least expected. There is new evidence suggesting that children's health may be compromised by one of the most popular warm weather activities. Recreational fountains are an increasingly attractive activity for children, and these fountains are often prominent features of shopping areas and amusement parks. The fountains give kids the opportunity to cool off on hot days and have fun while caregivers can relax. One enticing feature of these fountains includes water that shoots out of the ground in a timed sequence. If you have ever watched kids playing in one of these fountains, you know that there is sheer delight as kids are surprised by where the water will come from next.

Most of these fountains recirculate their water, meaning that the water drains into a basin under the fountain and is continuously reused in the fountain. In some ways this is similar to a public pool, except that the water is spraying rather than remaining stationary. Similar to a pool, the water must be chlorinated to ensure that microbiological organisms are kept under control. This is especially important with fountains because kids love to stand directly over the jets, a practice that could lead to rinsing fecal bacteria and viruses from the child. These potential pathogens then go into the basin under the fountain and, if not properly treated, will recirculate to the next child who comes in contact with the water.

This recreational fountain scenario played out in 2002 in The Netherlands.[10] Almost 200 school-aged children played in a fountain during a class outing and about 100 of these kids developed symptoms associated with foodborne illness within two days of the outing. Researchers surveyed the kids and their adult caregivers and narrowed the source down to either the fountain water or ice cream that many of the kids ate that day. After analyzing stool samples and conducting an environmental investigation, they discovered that the culprit for the illness was a norovirus and that the water in the fountain was the source of the virus. As children played in the fountain, they got the water in their mouths and could have directly ingested the virus. Other children could have had the virus on their skin and ingested it when they ate without washing their hands—after all, who needs to wash up when you have been playing in a fountain?

Water, food, and personal hygiene issues come together in disaster situations such as floods, tornadoes, and hurricanes. Major disasters can cripple all sanitation measures including drinking water, wastewater, and food safety. Hurricane Katrina was an historical event that will be remembered for images of people stranded on their roofs, massive destruction to legendary neighborhoods, and an ineffective response from Washington, D.C. Hurricane Katrina could also be remembered for the gastrointestinal illness that thousands of evacuees from New Orleans experienced while in temporary shelters. According to the CDC, more than 6,500 evacuees reported acute stomach distress, including diarrhea and vomiting, during the 10-day period of September 2–12, 2005.[11] Stool samples confirmed that the cause of the illness was a norovirus.

Perhaps the most alarming characteristic of the Katrina outbreak was that police and rescue personnel were also ill, suggesting that the virus was spreading from contact with evacuees and perhaps even inanimate objects. Public health response in disasters is a critical component of the overall response team. Imagine the responders who are there to help being as sick as the victims and you can envision a major problem as a result of this virus.

Norovirus knows no boundaries. It has come to the point where we should probably label the virus as endemic because it is always present in low levels in the population. It shows up in food, in water, and during critical emergencies. It has also been a major problem for people who are looking to have some fun on vacation.

LET'S TAKE A CRUISE

Noroviruses are perhaps best known for the impact that they have had on the cruise ship industry. Cruise ships offer a wonderful environment in which to share pathogens. There is food available all the time, there are lots of water-related activities, strangers live in close contact with one another, and people come from all over the world to take a cruise. There has probably always been some history of gastrointestinal illnesses on cruise ships, but in recent years, the reported incidence and number of people sickened has increased.

Passengers who have been on a cruise that was involved in an outbreak of the virus tell stories of being treated like prisoners, confined to their rooms and not allowed to touch any food with their hands.[12] Staff on these ships, wearing face masks and gloves and carrying spray bottles of high-powered sanitizer, also create an alarming picture that is sure to unsettle passengers. The norovirus can turn the dream vacation into an unforgettable nightmare.

The CDC requires cruise ships to report cases of illness to their Vessel Sanitation Program (VSP). The number of reports coming from cruise ships has been rising rapidly since 1994. Based on data available on the Web site of the VSP, the number of reported outbreaks increased from 1994 to 2007. In 1994, there were 5 documented outbreaks on cruise ships; by 2007 there were more than 35. The number of outbreaks reported increased the most dramatically from 2001 to 2002—from 4 in 2001 to more than 20 in 2002. It is possible that these increases could be the result of enhanced surveillance and media coverage of outbreaks, but it still paints a picture of a growing problem.

While the number of outbreaks may seem small—36 outbreaks in hundreds of cruises—the number of people sickened in each outbreak is not insignificant. For example, one outbreak aboard a Carnival Cruise Lines ship in November 2006 involved 536 passengers and 143 crew members; almost 20 percent of the passengers and 12 percent of the crew were ill on this cruise. Overall, reports filed by cruise lines and available on the VSP Web site indicate that, since 2004, more than 11,000 passengers of cruise ships have reported symptoms of gastrointestinal illness. This amounts to about 5 percent of all passengers who were on board the ships involved in the outbreaks. Basing estimates on the total number of passengers on the ships with the illness, if you take a cruise your risk of spending your vacation on the toilet with diarrhea and vomiting is somewhere in the neighborhood of one in 20. Don't expect to see this featured in any cruise advertisements.

One of the passengers on the Carnival cruise in November 2006 was David Lee Fitzgerald, a 76-year-old retired United Airlines worker. Mr. Fitzgerald was on the cruise with his wife and several family members. According to news accounts, he got sick about four days into the trip. His wife was sick as well, but had recovered by the time he started showing symptoms. He was treated by the ship's doctor, but he could not shake the diarrhea and vomiting. He became severely dehydrated and he died on board the ship six days after the symptoms started. Despite Carnival Cruise Lines's assertion and the Broward medical examiner's confirmation that Mr. Fitzgerald died from preexisting conditions, in October 2007, his widow filed a lawsuit against the ship and its physician.[13]

Other norovirus outbreaks on cruise ships include one in January 2007 on the *Queen Elizabeth 2 (QE2)*, one of the most renowned ships in operation today. During this outbreak almost 300 passengers and 30 crew members were sick, amounting to about 17 percent of all of those on board.

The final outbreak in 2007 was onboard the *Pride of Hawaii*, which is operated by Norwegian Cruise Lines. About 150 passengers and crew, or 6 percent of all of those on the ship, were sick with vomiting and diarrhea. Anyone who had symptoms was quarantined in their cabin for at least 24 hours, but the illness was still able to spread.

Ensuring Safe Passage

The VSP is responsible for inspecting cruise ships to ensure a safe and healthy environment for passengers and workers. In 2007, the VSP conducted more than 200 inspections, some of which were repeat inspections on the same vessel. For example, the *QE2* that was involved in the first reported norovirus outbreak in 2007 was inspected three times in 2007 and did not fail any of these inspections.

Ships are evaluated on a 100-point scale using the 2005 *Vessel Sanitation Program Operations Manual.*[14] The VSP is responsible for inspecting all vessels that "have a foreign itinerary, call on a U.S. port, and carry thirteen or more passengers." The main focus of the inspection is food safety and environmental health. Inspectors evaluate drinking water, pools and spas, pest management, child-care centers, and overall basic sanitation procedures. Each vessel receives a score based on the inspection results, with the perfect score being 100. If a vessel receives a score of 85 or below, it is considered unsatisfactory. Of the more than 200 inspections in 2007, only three vessels received scores of 85 or below. This suggests that the problem of norovirus on cruise ships is most likely a people problem; that is, the virus is "welcomed" aboard the ship the same time as the passengers are.

The VSP is also responsible for outbreak investigation and management on board vessels during a cruise. Ships are supposed to keep a log of reported gastrointestinal illness, and if the number of reported illnesses exceeds 2 percent of those on board, the VSP is supposed to be notified. This notification is not mandatory however, and it is probably in the cruise line's interest to keep these types of outbreaks as low profile as possible. Considering the number of people who take cruises every year, the problem might get worse before it gets better.

According to the Cruise Lines International Association (CLIA), the number of passengers who have taken cruises has more than doubled since 1995. In 1995, an estimated 4,721,000 people took cruises worldwide.[15] This number jumped to about 12 million by 2006, almost a 40 percent increase. While there are more opportunities for cruising now than in 1995, some of the increase is also accounted for by the larger size of newer ships, with more capacity for passengers than ever before.

CLIA comprises 19 of the largest cruise lines in the world including American, Carnival, Holland America, Norwegian, Princess, and Royal Caribbean. According to the CLIA, its member cruise lines added seven new vessels between 2004 and 2006, growing from 144 ships to 151 ships. This constituted an 8 percent change in the number of berths available between 2005 and 2006. Furthermore, as many as 26 new cruise ships are expected to join the current North American fleet by the year 2010. The CLIA estimates that more than 31 million North Americans will take a cruise sometime between 2007 and 2010. The average ship holds about 2,000 passengers, so if 12 million people took cruises during 2006, this means that more than 5,000 cruises set sail during the year.

While the cruise industry is thriving and has the potential to grow, the government agency responsible for environmental health and safety on the cruises is shrinking. The VSP is part of the National Center for Environmental Health at the CDC. The budget for environmental health and injury at the CDC for the year 2007 was almost 4 percent lower than the 2006 budget. In addition, the line items specified as "environmental health activities" in the category of environmental health and injury incurred a 15 percent decrease in 2007 from 2006 budget figures. So, while the need for additional environmental health inspectors to monitor cruise ships keeps growing, the availability of these inspectors, and the entire inspection program, is in jeopardy of being budgeted right out of the government.

The median age for those who take cruises is 49, and a high percentage of the passengers are retired, indicating a significant numbers of passengers are over 60. Noroviruses must love taking cruises because a ship creates an almost perfect environment for their survival. On a cruise, the virus has a captive group of susceptible hosts who are able to share the virus quite effectively with each other. Also available are a multitude of other vehicles that can transmit the virus to a host including buffets, spas, and swimming pools. For this reason, cruises have probably always had relatively high rates of infectious diseases, especially those related to the stomach, but the scale of the infections has gotten larger in recent years. Some cruise lines have cut trips short, others have cancelled cruises altogether, all because of the smallest organism known to humankind: the virus.

TARGETING THE ELDERLY

One factor that contributes to the severity of viral disease is the susceptibility of the host that is infected. This is why viruses can be especially dangerous to the elderly, children, or anyone with a preexisting medical condition. It is likely that many more people on cruise ships have received a dose of the virus, but if they were healthy, they may have not experienced any symptoms. Viruses prey on people who are already weak or have compromised immune systems because of preexisting conditions, such as AIDS; age is also considered a major factor in susceptibility. This is the reason why it is so critical for people over the age of 50 to get an influenza vaccine every year. Influenza is caused by a virus and healthy, younger people can usually withstand a case of the flu without major complications; this is not necessarily the case with people over 50.

Norovirus obtained during the cruise may never be implicated as the cause of Mr. Fitzgerald's death as discussed previously. However, in 2006, the first death in the United States in which norovirus was identified as the cause of death was reported in North Carolina. A 90-year old woman in a long-term care facility died from acute gastroenteritis.[16] This patient suffered from diarrhea and dehydration for three days before she died; the cause of death listed on the certificate was gastroenteritis. This is a unique situation because death records do not usually identify infectious disease as the cause of death. Rather, death certificates will note heart or kidney failure as the causal factors, even if the person had an underlying chronic condition such as cancer. It is especially challenging when recording the deaths of the elderly because there could be many factors that contribute to the mortality, so for the physician to note gastroenteritis as the cause indicates that it was the chief factor in the death.

Long-term care facilities are dangerous places when it comes to the spread of infectious disease, especially noroviruses. Almost one-half of the outbreaks of norovirus in 2006 occurred in long-term care facilities, and a significant percentage of these events are caused by ill food service workers in these facilities. It may be difficult to believe, but it is a never-ending battle to ensure that health care workers are conscientious hand washers. Some facilities have taken steps to make it easier for workers by including hand sanitizers in convenient locations and offering incentives for hand washing. Nevertheless, outbreaks of viral illness in long-term care facilities have been rising in recent years. An example from one state paints the picture as, according to CDC, there were 17 outbreaks of acute gastroenteritis in long-term care facilities in North Carolina in 2006. These outbreaks involved at least 573 residents and 288 staff members. This is an increase from six outbreaks in North Carolina in 2005 and three in 2004. It is likely that norovirus played a significant role in these outbreaks.

If the situation in North Carolina with the increasing numbers of acute gastroenteritis outbreaks is of concern, then the situation in Wisconsin should be downright alarming. In 2006 Wisconsin reported 206 outbreaks to CDC, up from only 23 in 2005. Perhaps more importantly, 78 percent of the outbreaks of AGE occurred in long-term care facilities. More than 2,000 people either living in or working for long-term care facilities in Wisconsin were ill during 2006. Two people died, but unlike the North Carolina case, the cause of death was not identified as gastroenteritis even though the people who died were suffering from it.

Similar situations in long-term care facilities have occurred across the country. Not only has there been a tremendous increase in the reported number of outbreaks of AGE during 2005 and 2006, but the number being reported in long-term care facilities accounts for almost 60 percent of these outbreaks. Norovirus as the confirmed cause of the reported illnesses accounts for almost 30 percent of the cases. While the 30 percent figure is considered a reliable estimate, it is likely that noroviruses are the cause of a much higher percentage of illness because many of reported outbreaks are caused by unknown and unconfirmed sources. Because conditions in a long-term care facility are so conducive to the spread of viruses, it may be that the cases of stomach illness in such facilities are more likely to be related to viruses than bacteria.

One reason that long-term care facilities are prone to the spread of norovirus is the same reason that illness spreads in other institutional settings, such as child development centers. That is, people who work in long-term care facilities are often hourly employees who are underpaid and overworked. According to the Bureau of Labor Statistics (BLS), there were 1,375,000 nurse's aides, orderlies, and attendants in long-term care facilities in 2004. This staff is responsible for direct care of patients, including helping with routine personal hygiene needs. The educational requirements for many of the direct-care personnel include 75 hours of training for nurse's aides; orderlies and attendants generally do not even need a high school diploma to do this kind of work. Perhaps some training in basic microbiology is needed to curtail the spread of disease in these facilities.

ONE HEARTY VIRUS

Noroviruses are a leading cause of diarrhea because they are hearty viruses that can survive for extended periods of time in the environment. They have the capability to survive in water that has been treated with chlorine at levels that would be adequate to disinfect water from most other pathogens. When someone with the virus vomits, more than 30 million virus particles can be released, and as few as 10 virus particles can make someone sick.[17] Even though the major route of transmission is fecal-oral, there is evidence emerging that virus particles can become airborne during an outbreak.[18] The first study to show the possibility of airborne transmission took place in the United Kingdom after a dinner at a hotel in December 1998.[19] During the meal, one of the guests vomited on the floor. The vomit was quickly cleaned up, and the dinner proceeded.

Three days after the episode in the hotel, some of the diners who attended the event contacted environmental health officials to report that they were ill with diarrhea and vomiting. The environmental health professionals conducted a complete investigation and could find no evidence that the virus was transmitted via the food served at the event. None of the staff reported being ill and people who had eaten in the part of the hotel in which the women did not vomit were not sick. The researchers concluded that this was a case in which virus particles were emitted into the air as the woman vomited. The particles must have become airborne and settled on food and surfaces that led to some of the nearby diners ingesting them and ultimately becoming ill. The mere proximity of diners to the vomiting woman led to sickness; the woman never had to touch anything that they ate.

Once the virus is introduced into the environment, it is patient and waits for a living host to pick it up and offer it a place to thrive. Remember that viruses cannot reproduce without a living host and will eventually die without cells to invade. So the best way to stop the spread of viruses is to prevent them from infecting a host in the first place. This requires vigilant personal hygiene and, when this measure fails, the environment must be decontaminated. In December 2007, an elementary school in British Columbia cancelled classes because more than 25 percent of their students were sick with norovirus. The school was triple-sanitized before the kids came back, a much more resource-intensive prevention method than good hand washing. Cruise ships and other facilities also undergo such rigorous scrubbings after outbreaks.

Despite our increasing understanding of the spread of norovirus and a media emphasis on the disease, the CDC has confirmed that the number of outbreaks of noroviruses has risen since 2003. In addition, new strains of the virus are emerging. Our food supply continues to be a good vehicle for transmitting this virus, but the virus has to get on the food from an infected person. This makes dealing with the virus all the more challenging because it is impossible to legislate and enforce good hand washing practices.

NOTES

1. James M. Jay, *Modern Food Microbiology*. 6th ed. (Gaithersburg, MD: Aspen, 2000).

2. L. R. Haaheim, J. R. Pattison, and Richard J. Whitley, eds., *A Practical Guide to Clinical Virology* (Chichester, NY: John Wiley & Sons, 2002), http://www.library.ohiou.edu:2326/Details.aspx (accessed January 9, 2008).

3. World Health Organization, *Global Polio Eradication Initiative: The History,* http://www.polioeradication.org/history.asp#1789 (accessed January 10, 2008).

4. Friedrich Loeffler and P. Frosch. "Berichte der Kommission zur Erforschung der Maul- und Klauenseuche bei dem Institut fur Infektionskrankheiten," in *Milestones in Microbiology:1556 to 1940,* transl. and ed. by Thomas D. Brock (Washington, D.C.: ASM Press, 1998), 149.

5. Rudolf Rott and Stuart Siddell, "One Hundred Years of Animal Virology," *Journal of General Virology* 79 (1998): 2871–74.

6. All outbreaks are taken from common news sources.

7. All of the outbreaks discussed in this chapter are real-life examples provided by environmental health professionals during an online survey from August to September 2007.

8. CDC, "Norovirus Activity—United States, 2006–2007," *Morbidity and Mortality Weekly Reports* 56 (2007): 842–46, http://www.cdc.gov/mmwr/preview/mmwrhtml/mm5633a2.htm.

9. CDC, "Multisite Outbreak of Norovirus Associated with a Franchise Restaurant—Kent County, Michigan, May 2005," *Morbidity and Mortality Weekly Reports* 55 (2006): 395–97, http://www.cdc.gov/mmwr/preview/mmwrhtml/mm5514a3.htm.

10. Christian J. P.A. Hoebe et al., "Norovirus Outbreak among Primary Schoolchildren Who Had Played in a Recreational Water Fountain," *Journal of Infectious Diseases* 189 (2004): 699–705.

11. CDC, "Norovirus Outbreak among Evacuees from Hurricane Katrina—Houston, Texas, September, 2005," *Morbidity and Mortality Weekly Reports* 54, no. 40 (2005): 1016–18, http://www.cdc.gov/mmwr/preview/mmwrhtml/mm5440a3.htm.

12. Patrick Healy, "Tormented by Viral Stowaway, Cruise Ship Staggers into Port," *New York Times,* September 3, 2005, B1.

13. Martha Brannigan, "Widow Sues Carnival Alleging Wrongful Death," *The Miami Herald,* October 26, 2006, Business and Financial News, p. 3C.

14. CDC, *Vessel Sanitation Operations Manual* (2005), http://www.cdc.gov/nceh/vsp/operationsmanual/OPSManual2005.pdf.

15. CLIA, *The Cruise Industry, 2006 Economic Summary* (2006), http://www.cruising.org/press/research/2006.CLIA.EconomicSummary.pdf.

16. CDC, "Norovirus Activity—United States, 2006–2007," http://www.cdc.gov/mmwr/preview/mmwrhtml/mm5633a2.htm.

17. Shabin S. Nanji, "Cruise Ships, Oysters, and Edible Vaccines: Revisiting the Non-cultivable Norwalk-Like Virus Responsible for Outbreaks of Gastroenteritis," *Clinical Microbiology Newsletter* 26 (2004): 1–4.

18. CDC, "Norwalk-Like Viruses: Public Health Consequences and Outbreak Management," *Morbidity and Mortality Weekly Reports* 50, no. RR09 (2001), http://www.cdc.gov/mmwr/preview/mmwrhtml/rr5009a1.htm.

19. P. J. Marks et al., "Evidence for Airborne Transmission of Norwalk-Like Virus in a Hotel Restaurant," *Epidemiology and Infection* 124 (2000): 481–87.

— 5 —

There Is Something in the Water

Water is an integral part of food safety. It enters the food supply in fish, processed foods, ice, produce, and drinking water. With this in mind, the safety of the world's water supply is critical to keeping our food supply safe. Waterborne disease outbreaks occur on a regular basis, but we usually associate these with developing countries that lack adequate sanitation. However, the countries that have state-of-the-art sanitation systems can no longer ignore the condition of water in developing countries. As we increase our imports of such water-reliant foods as seafood and fresh produce, water from across the globe can be brought directly into our homes.

CONTAMINATED WATER—FROM GLOBAL TO LOCAL

Diseases that are caused by drinking contaminated water are the result of many factors, most of which are human-induced. One characteristic of waterborne pathogens is that they discriminate based on the wealth of the population . People who live in poverty are more likely to suffer from infectious diseases resulting from consuming drinking water contaminated with microbiological pathogens than those populations who are wealthier. This is one reason why the poorest countries in the world have the highest rates of diseases such as cholera and dysentery—both bacterial diseases that are caused by direct exposure to polluted water. Countries with the lowest poverty rates are less likely to be directly exposed to organisms in drinking water; rather there is a secondary exposure in food. However, even in countries with adequate water sanitation, there are still pockets of poverty that contain unsafe drinking water.

Producing clean drinking water is expensive. Sometimes it requires more than just drilling a deeper well. It may mean that technology needs to be installed to treat water using chemical disinfectants to eradicate microbes. Modern drinking water systems include several mechanical steps to disinfect the water and ensure that it is aesthetically appealing. Drinking water treatment is based on the assumption that all water is contaminated and must be sanitized to ensure that it is safe when it reaches the tap.

In the United States, public drinking water comes from both surface and ground water sources. If a system serves more than 25 people, or includes 15 connections, for at least 60 days per year, the water must comply with drinking water standards. The government sets maximum contaminant levels for chemicals, radionuclides, and microbiological organisms that are permitted in drinking water at the tap. In order to control the levels of bacteria and viruses, public drinking water is usually treated at facilities that disinfect the water with chlorine or some other proven sanitation method.

Private drinking water systems are generally wells and other sources that provide water to residences. These systems are common in rural areas in the United States and other developed countries mainly due to the expense of installing distribution systems far from public treatment plants. Private systems are essentially unregulated by the government; it is up to the owner of the system to ensure the water is safe to drink. This means that people who have wells on their own properties are responsible to have their wells tested for possible contamination on a regular basis. Testing drinking water is not something that many homeowners do and I am a case in point. The source of drinking water in my home is a private well, I am an environmental health professional and I understand the importance of regular well testing, but I can not remember the last time I had my own drinking water tested. In addition to access to clean drinking water, there is a relationship between wastewater treatment and safe drinking water that cannot be overlooked. If human waste is being dumped into the environment untreated, it is possible that infectious agents will make their way into the drinking water supply. As with public drinking water systems, wastewater management is expensive, requiring sewage collection systems in addition to treatment capabilities.

The regions in the world that have endemic infectious diseases are also the areas that do not have the current capacity for water treatment. The lack of clean drinking water translates into the lack of clean water for personal hygiene and cooking. When people wash their hands and cook with water that is contaminated with microbiological organisms, infectious disease will spread. We see the clear relationship between personal hygiene and food-borne diseases with both viral and bacterial pathogens and this relationship has been known for a very long time.

More than 100 years ago, the association between human waste and water-borne diseases was a controversial topic, but there were some who attempted to educate the public about the possible connection. For example, the controversy was portrayed in Henrik Ibsen's 1882 play *Enemy of the People*, which is the story of a doctor who believes that the thriving spa industry is making people sick. The play is a commentary on political forces that affect public health. It is also evidence of the challenges faced by those concerned with the public health ramifications of environmental contamination. It is obvious to us today that dirty water can make you sick, but historically, it has never been easy for public health pioneers to convince decision makers to commit the resources to address this, and other, environmental health problems.

The Human Waste–Drinking Water Connection Revealed

Imagine London, England, in the 1800s. People got their drinking water from common well pumps located throughout the city. The wastewater management system at this time consisted of dumping human waste in the streets. In one neighborhood, there was a lingering outbreak of diarrhea. One physician was curious as to why diarrhea was a serious problem in only one specific area of the city, considering that environmental conditions throughout the city were more or less the same. He suspected that there might be something in the water that people in this one neighborhood were drinking.

This physician was John Snow, and the well-known story of his investigation into the cause of the diarrhea in London is one of the pivotal moments in public health intervention and disease prevention.[1] One of the first things Snow did was plot the cases of diarrhea on a map to see if he could identify some exposure that the sick people might have in common. Upon examining the map, he suspected that one well pump was the source of some sort of organism that was making people sick. After he convinced city officials to remove the handle from the pump so people couldn't drink the water, the cases of diarrhea almost immediately diminished.

The cause of the diarrhea in London in the 1800s, the *Vibrio cholerae* bacteria, is still a major cause of diarrhea across the globe today. Until recently, John Snow and Robert Koch, who won the Nobel Prize for Medicine in 1905, were the two names linked to the discovery of the cholera bacteria.

However, another man alive at the same time was recently recognized as the scientist who truly identified the organism that causes cholera.

Filippo Pacini was an Italian doctor who was born to a cobbler in 1812. According to scant biographical accounts, he was a poor man whose research into the cause of human disease was essentially self-funded. He was in Florence, Italy, in 1854 when the city was in the midst of a cholera epidemic. As he performed autopsies on cholera victims, he recorded finding organisms in their intestines that he called vibrions. A vibrion is a motile bacterium, meaning that it has the ability to move on its own with the use of flagella.

Pacini took excellent notes and published an account of his discovery, but when John Snow and Robert Koch were investigating cholera, they were not aware of Pacini's work. In addition, much like the protagonist in the Ibsen play, Pacini could not convince the influential people in Italy that cholera was contagious and could be spread from person to person.[2] The result of Pacini's inability to raise awareness of the bacteria was that until 1965, the famed bacteriologist Robert Koch was credited with discovering the *Vibrio* bacteria that was identified as the cause of cholera. However, in 1965, Pacini was given the credit he deserved when an international committee responsible for classifying and naming bacteria replaced the Koch name with Pacini so that the bacteria is now known as *Vibrio cholerae Pacini*.

Back in England, John Snow concluded that water was the source of cholera bacteria and his observations and study of disease were the precursors to modern epidemiology. In addition, his findings about the connection between cholera bacteria and disease are the basis of what we know to be true today. Because of his research that uncovered this relationship, we know that the availability of clean drinking water is the critical element preventing the spread of this disease in modern times. Cholera is not a disease that is commonly found in countries like England or the United States in the twenty-first century. Even though there are confirmed cases in developed countries almost every year, they are almost always imported by travelers returning from regions with endemic levels of the disease.

On the other hand, outside of the developed countries, the WHO is concerned about the increasing incidence of cholera. The WHO reported that the number of reported cases of cholera in 2005 increased by approximately 20 percent over the 2004 numbers.[3] While the incidence of the disease is still highest in developing regions, especially West Africa, increasing incidence of cholera has the potential to become one of the major global public health and economic problems of our time because of international trade and travel. For example, according to the WHO, an outbreak of cholera in the early 1990s caused severe economic consequences in Peru as countries such as the United States refused to import food from them during the outbreak.

Relative to Cholera

Cholera is one of the *Vibrio* genus of bacteria, which consists of at least 80 different species. While cholera is an ancient pathogen, there are species of *Vibrio* that are still emerging, and some of these species have the capability to cause human disease. Contemporary research related to *Vibrio* is dynamic; new species are still being discovered, and there are scientists who have dedicated most of their professional research to classifying these bacteria. In November 2005, the Association of *Vibrio* Biologists was formed (www.vibriobiology.net), and a *Vibrio* 2007 conference was held in Paris in late November 2007. Despite all of the attention to *Vibrio* research, there are still numerous uncertainties surrounding these bacteria especially with respect to the most effective way to detect them in the environment, and how to best minimize their growth in harvested seafood.[4]

Even though *Vibrio* research is still evolving and it emerged as a pathogen in water in the late 1800s, we have known about the cholera pathogen, *Vibrio cholerae*, for thousands of years. There are historical records suggesting that cholera was the cause of illness as far back as the fifth century B.C.[5] On the other hand, the *Vibrio* bacteria that are of concern today, because of their ability to contaminate seafood, are relative newcomers to the infectious disease scene. One of these newcomers is *Vibrio parahaemolyticus*, a natural bacterium found in coastal water. It can survive in saltwater and generally thrives as water warms up, such as during the summer months.

Water temperature has been considered a critical element in the prevalence of this bacterium. This has led to the belief that the years when coastal waters are warmest for the longest periods of time will generally lead to higher levels of *V. parahaemolyticus* in coastal waters, translating into higher levels in seafood. The water temperature–bacteria population correlation suggests that the public health burden of illness associated with eating fish will increase as global temperatures rise. In addition, new research suggests that there may be other critical factors that affect the levels of *V. parahaemolyticus* in water, including salinity.[6] Furthermore, it may not be accurate to use measured levels of the bacteria in water as an indicator of seafood contamination because oysters may actually contain higher numbers of human disease-causing bacteria than the surrounding water does.

Because these bacteria are everywhere in the natural environment of coastal waters, they are almost always found in fresh seafood. The most common way in which people become sick from *V. parahaemolyticus* is from eating shellfish, in particular raw shellfish such as oysters and clams. Because they thrive in warm-water habitats, U.S. outbreaks are often linked to shellfish harvested in Gulf Coast waters, such as Mississippi and Alabama. On the other hand, there are new data that are raising concerns about the spread of these bacteria in coastal waters in geographic areas that are normally cooler.

In 2005 an outbreak on a cruise ship in Alaska was connected to oysters that were farmed in Alaskan waters. This was a notable outbreak because it was the first time *V. parahaemolyticus* was documented so far north.[7] Another outbreak occurred in 2006, when there were cases of diarrhea in several states including New York, Washington, and Oregon. The CDC was able to trace the source of the illnesses to oysters and clams that were harvested in the Pacific Northwest and shipped to restaurants throughout the country.

When a person eats seafood contaminated with *V. parahaemolyticus*, diarrhea may begin in as little as four hours after the meal, with the average time being about 15 hours. In most cases the victim will recover in a short period of time, about two days. But in some instances hospitalization may be required to deal with dehydration. Because the infection is generally mild and sporadic, most public health professionals both at the local level and globally believe that the incidence is greatly underreported. There may be even larger outbreaks that are not reported to global health authorities for fear that travel to some destinations would be curtailed if people were alarmed about consuming regional seafood.

Minimizing Oyster Illness

As long as there is a demand for raw oysters, *V. parahaemolyticus* will remain a public health risk. Risks from shellfish were recognized by the federal government in the early 1900s and, in response to the Surgeon General's request in 1925, the National Shellfish Sanitation Program (NSSP) was born. The NSSP focused on the role of the states in ensuring that shellfish is safe for human consumption. The federal government, in the form of the Public Health Service, was made responsible for providing assistance to the states. The Public Health Service also certifies that states are properly overseeing shellfish harvesting and processing according to acceptable sanitary standards.

Under the NSSP, state governments can develop their own regulations and controls to monitor the shellfish industry. In 1975, the NSSP attempted to develop national regulations, but this effort went nowhere due to unfavorable comments on the draft regulation. Today, the NSSP remains an organization that offers only guidance to states and industries regarding shell-fish practices to minimize public health risks. Participation in the NSSP is still voluntary, and the federal government has no enforcement authority if states do not follow their guidance.

Ultimately, in a familiar story, the risk of consuming raw shellfish is in the hands of consumers. One of the best ways for consumers to minimize their risk of this illness is to be sure that oysters are purchased from reputable sources. A listing of firms that ship shellfish that are certified as meeting international sanitation guidelines is updated monthly and available online from the federal government (http://vm.cfsan.fda.gov/~ear/shellfis.html). When purchasing any fresh seafood, but especially shellfish that will be con-sumed without cooking, it is important to look for fish that is on ice. The best way to inhibit the growth of dangerous bacteria in shellfish is to keep the product cold enough, and out of the temperature danger zone.

In 1982, the Interstate Shellfish Sanitation Conference (ISSC) was formed for the purpose of enhancing the safety of shellfish in the United States. ISSC is another voluntary organization comprising representatives from the shellfish industry, states that have an interest in shellfish production, and the federal government, including the FDA and the Environmental Protection Agency (EPA). There are three task forces within the ISSC that make rec-ommendations to the entire conference. These recommendations are voted on by the conference membership and are passed on to agencies that moni-tor shellfish production. According to the ISSC's Web site (www.issc.org), oysters are safe to eat if they are "harvested from approved waters, packed under sanitary conditions, and properly refrigerated." However, people with preexisting medical conditions such as liver disease, diabetes, or AIDS are advised to stay away from eating raw oysters.

Aside from guidance from the NSSP, lists for consumers, and an inter-state workgroup, the major approach that the government uses to address the issue of seafood safety is to require all seafood producers to employ the Haz-ard Analysis Critical Control Point system, also known as HACCP. This system essentially requires the processor to monitor the product from the time that he or she purchases it to the time it is at the retail establishment. The seafood processor identifies the critical points along the production line that could lead to dangerous conditions that might support microbio-logical growth. While this system is especially designed for processors who are freezing or cooking seafood for retail consumption, it can also work for seafood products that will be consumed raw.

According to the HACCP system, an example of a critical point in the process might be the time that it takes to get oysters from the loading dock into refrigeration. The processor would identify specific actions to take to ensure that this time period is minimized, and steps to take if the actions are not followed. For HACCP to work best with raw seafood the product has to be processed; this is often not the case as fresh seafood is often purchased right from the fishing boats that bring it onto the dock and then taken to the retail point of sale. There is no way that the government is able to ensure that all of the vessels that are licensed for harvesting and selling fresh seafood are following HACCP procedures. This means it is up to the consumer to be sure that the fish is coming from clean water and has been properly iced since it was caught. How many consumers are able to do this?

The HACCP system has been proven to be valid and effective at controlling microbiological hazards in numerous venues, but seafood processing might not be one of them. In 2001, the Government Accounting Office (GAO) produced a report entitled, "Federal Oversight of Seafood Does Not Sufficiently Protect Consumers." This report evaluated the efforts made by the FDA since they required seafood processors to employ HACCP in 1997. In the report, the GAO is very critical of the way in which the FDA has implemented the HACCP system. Four years after HACCP became mandatory for shellfish processors, less than one-half of the seafood processors in the country were using HACCP, and the FDA does not have the resources to inspect or enforce the regulations.

Furthermore, there is minimal oversight with seafood that is being imported into the United States. Again, this is due to a lack of resources and the inability of the government to inspect all imported seafood. To deal with the lack of resources for inspection, the FDA essentially allows seafood to enter the country without an inspection if the source has a documented system like HACCP in place. However, validating that importing countries have comparable processes is not being completed by FDA. The bottom line from the GAO's perspective is that, in 2001, the FDA was not ensuring that the seafood consumed in the United States (produced both domestically and imported), was safe to eat. Seafood, like fruits and vegetables, is a healthy food, but also like fruits and vegetables, it can be dangerous if not produced, stored, and prepared safely.

Returning to oysters specifically, the FDA conducted a risk assessment focusing on the pathways that lead to contaminated oysters; this risk assessment took several years to complete and was published in 2005.[8] The purpose of the risk assessment was to enhance the understanding of the conditions that contribute to the growth of bacteria in oysters. In this assessment, the FDA explains that the raw oyster industry is variable based on geography. That is, not all oysters are harvested, shipped, and sold in the same way. For example, oysters harvested in Louisiana remain on loading docks for longer periods of time than those harvested in other Gulf Coast states.

In the risk assessment, the FDA used a model to predict the risk of getting sick from eating raw oysters. The model included many assumptions related to environmental and oyster handling conditions. Even though the risk of illness from eating raw oysters harvested in the United States is relatively low, the FDA's model predicted that the risk is highest for those people who consume oysters harvested off the coast of Louisiana. The FDA explains that there are not enough data regarding the levels of bacteria in oysters at the time of consumption, but higher levels at the time of harvest probably translate into even higher levels by the time people eat them. This leads to the conclusion that controls should be in place to ensure that oysters destined for raw consumption are iced and kept cold from harvest to table.

When thinking about how water can contaminate the food supply and cause illness, it is easy to see how seafood might be a suspect. But there are numerous other foods that can come into contact with contaminated water, including produce. Water for irrigation as well as cleaning can inoculate fresh fruits and vegetables with pathogens that will not be cooked any further before eating. This was the scenario that played out in Pennsylvania in 2003 when hundreds of people became ill from eating green onions.

CHIPS, SALSA, AND HEPATITIS

In November 2003, one of the largest documented outbreaks of hepatitis A in the United States occurred in Pennsylvania. Before this outbreak subsided more than 600 people were ill, three people died, and a major restaurant franchise that had previously filed for bankruptcy protection went out of business in the midst of a public relations nightmare.

The Fecal Hepatitis

Hepatitis is often thought of as a disease that is spread only through close contact such as kissing or sharing a needle. However hepatitis A (HAV) is the form of the virus that can be transmitted in food and water, and it is considered an important cause of viral foodborne infections. Although documented foodborne outbreaks of HAV are relatively rare in the United States, studies have shown that a significant percentage of food service workers may be carriers of the virus, leading to the suspicion that food-related cases may be underreported.[9]

There are five types of the hepatitis virus and they are labeled alphabetically as hepatitis A, B, C, D, and E. Of the five types, hepatitis A (HAV), B (HBV), and C (HCV) are the most common causes of illness. Of these three hepatitis viruses, it is HAV that is transmitted via the fecal-oral route and can therefore be spread in food and water. Both HBV and HCV require close personal contact for transmission, usually with blood, or with other bodily fluids such as saliva or semen.

The incidence of HAV has declined steadily in the United States since the early 1990s, when about 12 out of every 100,000 people could expect to be infected.[10] In 2005, the incidence of HAV had declined to about two per 100,000 people. The decline is largely the result of widespread vaccination that is especially targeted at children who live in states with high levels of HAV.

HAV is endemic in developing countries, and contrary to the way most endemic diseases operate in these countries, outbreaks of the disease are relatively rare. This is because people become immune to the illness once they contract it. So, in countries where HAV is ubiquitous in the environment, the population is exposed as children, giving them lifelong immunity. The WHO classifies countries by how endemic HAV is, or the "endemicity" of the disease.[11] Africa, parts of Asia, and Central and South America have very high levels of endemicity, meaning that the virus is always circulating in the environment. In these countries, the average age of a person with HAV is under five years old and HAV is usually acquired from direct contact with infected people or contaminated food and water.

Countries such as the United States, Canada, Australia, and Western Europe have low levels of endemicity. The age of infection can be as low as 5 years old and as high as 40 years old. Unlike countries with high endemicity, outbreaks occur more often and are usually tied to some common source. Since HAV is not endemic, it is often imported from other countries, either in food or with people. An outbreak in Canada in May 2005 offers an excellent example of how international travel can lead to an outbreak in a country that does not have endemic levels.[12] In this instance, a food service worker from Sri Lanka traveled home for a visit and when he returned to Canada he went back to work at a restaurant. Within a couple of weeks 16 people who had eaten at the restaurant were diagnosed with HAV. The environmental investigation of the restaurant uncovered poor sanitation techniques and a lack of awareness of appropriate hand washing methods; the Sri Lankan food service worker was not sick.

The Hepatitis Niche

All of the hepatitis viruses are classified in different families. The hepatitis A virus is in the picornavirus family, or Picornaviridae. This family contains the viruses that contribute the greatest burden to global infectious viral diseases: enteroviruses and rhinoviruses. Enteroviruses are those that cause gastrointestinal distress, while rhinoviruses are respiratory in nature. The term picornavirus is assembled from "pico," which means small, and "rna," meaning ribonucleic acid. Although HAV is a member of the Picornaviridae family, in which there are five genera, it is singled out as its own genus, "hepatovirus." Singling out hepatitis A as its own genus in the family is due to the fact that it only attacks liver cells, or hepatocytes.

Since the hepatitis virus attacks the liver, one of the symptoms it causes is jaundice, or a yellowing of the skin. Jaundice is caused by high levels of the chemical bilirubin in the blood. Bilirubin is a waste product that remains after red blood cells release iron into the blood. A normal liver will help the body eliminate bilirubin from the blood, causing stool to be brown. When the liver is unable to efficiently eliminate the bilirubin, the color of urine, feces, eyes, and skin changes to a yellowish color, so, jaundice is indicative of a problem in the liver. The first documented epidemic of jaundice is expected to have occurred in 1745 on the Mediterranean island of Minorca.[13]

The Mexican Virus

The most notable recent outbreak of hepatitis A in the United States occurred in fall 2003 in a suburb of Pittsburgh, Pennsylvania. The outbreak was brought to light by a concerned physician who reportedly contacted the Pennsylvania Department of Health on November 1, 2003, to report several cases of HAV; he thought this was unusual because he had only treated one case in the previous year.[14] It became evident that the one thing that the cases had in common was dining at the same Chi-Chi's restaurant. The health department immediately inspected the restaurant and did not find any environmental health violations, but learned that several food service workers were sick. Within 10 days more than 100 people were confirmed sick with HAV and the restaurant voluntarily closed.

While the media was focusing on the Pennsylvania situation, there were outbreaks of HAV occurring in other states. Tennessee, North Carolina, and Georgia were reporting outbreaks involving more than 400 people. Microbiologists studied the outbreaks in the other states and concluded that green onions were the likely source of the virus, even though the strains of the virus were not identical.[15] This led to the determination that there may have actually been several distinct outbreaks of HAV occurring in the fall of 2003, all linked to green onions from the same area of Mexico, but different in terms of the genetic makeup of the virus. Research such as this underscores the challenge in understanding both the biology and the means of how HAV spreads among people.

The HAV outbreak in 2003 was not the first time that green onions were implicated in a foodborne outbreak. In 1998, at least 48 people were confirmed infected with HAV in an Ohio community just northwest of Columbus. The investigation into the cause of the illnesses identified green onions served at one restaurant as the most probable cause of the outbreak.[16] The sources of the green onions in this outbreak were never determined but it is likely that they came from one of two farms in Mexico.

During the 2003 Pennsylvania outbreak, the FDA went to Mexico to inspect facilities that were exporting green onions into the United States. They discovered that it was not possible to obtain environmental samples, since it was December and green onions were not currently being harvested.[17] The inspectors were concerned however with unsanitary conditions at the processing facilities, inadequate personal hygiene of employees, the safety of the water used to irrigate the fields, and the ice that that was preserving fresh produce. The results of these inspections reinforce the difficulties that the U.S. government faces in ensuring the safety of food that is imported, especially from areas with endemic levels of infectious disease.

In late November of 2003, the Mexican government halted exports from four companies that were suspected to be the source of the hepatitis. This led to serious economic concerns on the part of the green onion farmers in Mexico and their ability to recover from the negative publicity surrounding the documented outbreaks. Meanwhile back in the United States, victims of the Pennsylvania outbreak were lining up attorneys to represent them in lawsuits against Chi-Chi's. In December 2005, Chi-Chi's bankruptcy was approved and part of the asset liquidation included settling more than 400 claims from hepatitis victims, for a total of somewhere between 9 and 12 million dollars.

Once the hepatitis outbreak faded into the background, green onions were again on the menus of restaurants all over the country. Consumers forgot about the HAV scare until 2006 when green onions once again emerged as the potential cause of another foodborne outbreak, this one caused by a bacteria that is known for making people sick from eating undercooked hamburgers. Taco Bell removed green onions from their restaurants in late 2006 after almost 100 people in northeastern United States were sickened by *E. coli* O157:H7. This time it was a California farm that was implicated as the source of the contaminated onions.

FOOD, WATER AND THE GEOGRAPHY OF DISEASE

Ironically, even though drinking water can be a source of *E. coli* O157:H7, it is arguably our demand for cheap meat that contributes to water contamination. There is little doubt that large-scale "factory farming" creates conditions that challenge the management of manure. In 2000, a small farming community in Walkerton, Ontario, demonstrated the ill effects that intensive animal farming can have on the safety of the water supply. There were numerous large feedlots in the community, and it is likely that manure made its way into the public drinking water supply for the community. More than 2,300 people were sickened by *E. coli* O157:H7 and seven people died, making this one of the worst public health disasters in Canada.[18]

One way to manage manure that is an acceptable practice in the United States is to apply the manure to cropland as fertilizer. Although estimates vary, one 1,000-pound cow can produce about 15 tons of manure a year, so a feedlot with 200 cows has the capacity to produce 3,000 tons, or about 6 million pounds of manure to dispose of every year. This creates a major waste management problem and leaves us with trillions of tons of manure to deal with every year—that's *trillions* of tons of manure. One solution to this problem is to use manure as a natural fertilizer to enhance agriculture, but there is some evidence that if the manure is contaminated with infectious agents, the crops can become contaminated as well. For example, one study found that if *E. coli* O157:H7 is present in manure it can stay in the soil for months, and end up making root vegetables such as carrots and onions unsafe to eat.[19]

Where you live can affect your probability of being sickened by pathogens associated with agriculture, especially pathogens causing waterborne diseases. Research in the western United States suggests that people who live in rural communities are more likely to be exposed to pathogens such as *E. coli* O157:H7 than those who live in more urban areas.[20] This geographic relationship may be related to public health infrastructure capabilities such as the availability of modern drinking water and wastewater systems. It could also be related to the probability of exposure to livestock that are natural carriers of many pathogens.

Direct and indirect contact with livestock is a factor in the spread of foodborne disease, and opportunities for this contact occur in settings such as zoos and fairs. Since 1991, there have been about 50 disease outbreaks in humans associated with exposure to animals in public settings.[21] People get sick after they touch animals or come in contact with areas that animals have infected, and they then enjoy some cotton candy or funnel cake. In many of these venues, hand washing facilities are marginal and nowhere near the livestock—a fact that contributes to the spread of disease. Studies have shown that during outbreaks linked with exposure to animals those who washed their hands were less likely to be sick.

NONBACTERIAL AND NONVIRAL,
THE OTHER PATHOGEN

The most talked about outbreak of waterborne disease in the United States occurred in the Milwaukee area in 1993. In a matter of a few days, pharmacists noticed that they could not keep antidiarrheal medications on their shelves. Suspecting that there was an outbreak of diarrhea occurring, public health officials were notified and thus began the investigation into an outbreak that made more than 400,000 people sick. The cause of the outbreak was not a bacteria or a virus. It was another of the food and waterborne pathogens, in the group known as parasites or protozoa.

The Parasites

The most common cause of diarrhea related to recreational swimming, *Cryptosporidium*, has also been a frequent cause of food-related disease outbreaks. According to the CDC, the incidence of cryptosporidiosis increased significantly from 2003 to 2005.[22] The increase in frequency is likely due to a combination of factors including increased awareness on the part of primary health care professionals, enhanced public attention to the illness because of some high-profile outbreaks, and greater public health surveillance activities.

The *Cryptosporidium* parasite was first described by Edward Tyzzer and reported in a two-page paper in 1907.[23] Interestingly, he discovered this parasite while working simultaneously on cancer research; he wasn't looking for the cause of waterborne diseases.[24] However, it wasn't until five years after his first description, in 1912, that the new genus of *Cryptosporidium parvum* was documented by Tyzzer in laboratory mice. For more than 60 years, Tyzzer's discovery was not given great weight by those who study human disease because this protozoan was not viewed as an important contributor to human illness. In the early 1980s, the public health and medical community stopped ignoring *C. parvum* as research emerged suggesting that this pathogen could indeed infect humans.

Tyzzer was described as a multifaceted researcher who was interested from an early age in the causes of animal disease. Tyzzer is perhaps most well known for his discovery of a disease in laboratory mice, caused by bacteria, that led to high fatality rates. This disease is now known as "Tyzzer's Disease" and remains an illness that is confined to animals rather than humans. He published his findings related to the mouse disease in 1917, one year after he succeeded Theobald Smith as the Chair of the Department of Comparative Pathology at Harvard. Tyzzer died at the age of 90 in 1965, but he left behind a legacy of research that has solidified his place as one of the most important parasitologists in history.

Eleven years after Tyzzer's death the *Cryptosporidium* parasite was documented for the first time in humans. Since then, it has been identified as a leading cause of waterborne disease and there have been several notable foodborne outbreaks. There is a combination of reasons why this parasite was not detected in humans for almost 70 years after it was first discovered in animals. As with many pathogens, especially *E. coli* O157:H7, social forces such as food consumption patterns are likely the major catalyst for the emergence of animal diseases in humans since the 1970s. Microbial pathogens that are common in the intestines of animals are now becoming common in water and food that we consume. Intensive agriculture and changing consumer preferences are arguably the most important factors in this jump from "farm to fork."[25]

Cryptosporidium Microbiology

Cryptosporidium is considered a protozoan parasite. It is an organism that can complete its entire complex lifecycle inside a host. While inside the host, *Cryptosporidium* develops oocysts, which are microscopic thick-walled vehicles that transport the zygote, or agent of reproduction, from host to host. Once the oocyst transfers the zygote to a host, reproduction will begin. The reproductive process of the parasite is what makes the host sick because the wall of the intestine is used as the platform. Oocysts are very efficient transportation mechanisms because they are resistant to many of the disinfection techniques that are commonly used to produce clean water and safe food, including chlorination.

There are 16 known species of *Cryptosporidium* and at least 33 different documented genotypes. The taxonomy of *Cryptosporidium* is still developing and genetic sequencing will likely help classify the parasite. There are numerous challenges that microbiologists face in identifying the parasite, and this is leading to difficulties in its classification.[26] It is known, however, that the species of the parasite that most commonly infects people through food and water is *C. parvum*.

Cryptosporidium can contaminate the food supply in numerous ways, including poor personal hygiene, food prepared with contaminated water, fresh produce contaminated directly by animal feces, and contaminated water for ice making.[27] Furthermore, it takes an extremely small amount of the pathogen to cause illness, and current methods for detecting the microbe in food and water are very limited. The most common route of exposure to this parasite is via water, and since conventional disinfection techniques do not work to kill this pathogen, infected water can subsequently contaminate food.

Cryptosporidiosis is the name of the illness that results from ingesting the parasite. The symptoms may begin anywhere from two to ten days after exposure and may include fever and abdominal cramps. Watery diarrhea may be mild in healthy people, but it can lead to dehydration in those who are weakened by another illness. Some people seem to recover from the illness only to find the symptoms flaring up again. Even after the symptoms are gone and the patient feels better, the *Cryptosporidium* oocysts will continue to be shed in the feces. This contributes to the spread of the disease, because people may let down their guard and stop paying attention to hand washing once their diarrhea subsides.

Even though this parasite has been a veterinary problem for some time, the first documented human cases of cryptosporidiosis occurred in 1976.[28] Since this is a disease that can be debilitating to those with compromised immune systems, as AIDS became more prevalent so did cryptosporidiosis. Cryptosporidiosis has become very common in AIDS patients and can be fatal to these immunocompromised individuals. In one documented case a patient visited a doctor to complain about watery diarrhea, only to be diagnosed with cryptosporidiosis as well as AIDS.[29]

THE MOST CHALLENGING FOOD MANAGEMENT ISSUE?

Water can be the source of numerous pathogens including viruses, bacteria, and parasites. Minimizing the impact of contaminated water on the food supply will require public health strategies that are international, regional, and local in nature. International efforts will be needed to ensure that imported seafood and produce from areas where waterborne diseases are endemic are safe for consumption anywhere.

Regional efforts, including those that are countrywide, will require a commitment to surveillance and rapid outbreak investigation. This is critical since the outbreaks that have occurred with the water–food connection have been shown to involve multiple states. At the local level, the best approach might be to focus on improving water supplies and wastewater sanitation. None of the approaches to improving water systems are inexpensive however, and it may be that the problem with parasites in our water supply will get worse before it gets better.

All of the efforts to break the chain of infection between water and food require resources and a political focus on the importance of environmental and public health. Sadly, this focus does not currently exist. The evidence is clear, and can be found in the numerous voluntary approaches that are our food safety net. If the history of environmental pollution has taught us anything, it is that those who are responsible for contaminating the environment are more likely to change their behaviors when it is required, rather than when it is merely an unenforceable suggestion.

NOTES

1. For example, UCLA has a Web site dedicated to John Snow and his work with cholera: http://www.ph.ucla.edu/epi/snow.html (accessed January 10, 2008).

2. Marina Bentivoglio and Paolo Pacini, "Filippo Pacini: A Determine Observer," *Brain Research Bulletin* 38, no. 2 (1995): 161–65.

3. WHO, "Cholera, 2005," *Weekly Epidemiological Record* 31 (2006): 297–308.

4. Yi-Cheng Su and Chengchu Liu, "*Vibrio parahaemolyticus:* A Concern for Seafood Safety," *Food Microbiology* 24 (2007): 549–58.

5. Maria Neira, "Cholera: A Challenge for the 21st Century," *World Health* 50 (1997): 9.

6. A. M. Zimmerman et al., "Variability of Total and Pathogenic *Vibrio parahaemolyticus* Densities in Northern Gulf of Mexico Water and Oysters," *Applied and Environmental Microbiology* 73, no. 23 (2007): 7589–96.

7. Joseph B. McLaughlin et al., "Outbreak of *Vibrio parahaemolyticus* Gastroenteritis Associated with Alaskan Oysters," *The New England Journal of Medicine* 353, no. 14 (2005): 1463–70.

8. FDA, *Quantitative Risk Assessment on the Public Health Impact of Vibrio parahaemolyticus in Raw Oysters* (2005), http://www.cfsan.fda.gov/%7Edms/vpra-toc.html (accessed January 10, 2008).

9. Anthony E. Fiore, "Hepatitis A Transmitted by Food," *Clinical Infectious Diseases* 38 (2004): 705–15.

10. Annemarie Wasley, Jeremy T. Miller, and Lyn Finelli, "Surveillance for Acute Viral Hepatitis—United States, 2005," *Morbidity and Mortality Weekly Report* 56, no. SS03 (2007): 1–24.

11. WHO, *Epidemic and Pandemic Alert and Response: Hepatitis A*, http://www.who.int/csr/disease/hepatitis/whocdscsredc2007/en/index4.html#worldwide (accessed January 10, 2008).

12. P. Heywood et al., "A Community Outbreak of Travel-Acquired Hepatitis A Transmitted by an Infected Food Handler," *Canada Communicable Disease Report* 1, no. 33 (2007): 16–23.

13. Jennifer A. Cuthbert, "Hepatitis A: Old and New," *Clinical Microbiology Reviews* 14, no. 1 (2001): 38–58.

14. C. Wheeler et al., "An Outbreak of Hepatitis A Associated with Green Onions," *New England Journal of Medicine* 353 (2005): 890–97.

15. J. J. Amon et al., "Molecular Epidemiology of Foodborne Hepatitis A Outbreaks in the United States, 2003," *The Journal of Infectious Diseases* 192 (2005): 1323–30.

16. Catherine M. Dentinger et al., "An Outbreak of Hepatitis A Associated with Green Onions," *The Journal of Infectious Diseases* 183 (2001): 1273–76.

17. FDA, "FDA Update on Recent Hepatitis A Outbreaks Associated with Green Onions from Mexico" (December 9, 2003), http://www.fda.gov/bbs/topics/NEWS/2003/NEW00993.html (accessed January 10, 2008).

18. S. Harris Ali, "A Socio-ecological Autopsy of the *E. coli O157:H7* Outbreak in Walkerton, Ontario, Canada," *Social Sciences & Medicine* 58 (2004): 2601–12.

19. Mahbub Islam et al., "Survival of *Escherichia coli* O157:H7 in Soil and on Carrots and Onions Grown in Fields Treated with Contaminated Manure Composts or Irrigated Water," *Food Microbiology* 22 (2005): 63–70.

20. Jason P. Haack et al., "*Escherichia coli* O157 Exposure in Wyoming and Seattle: Serologic Evidence of Rural Risk," *Emerging Infectious Diseases* 9, no. 10 (2003): 1226–31.

21. NCDC, "Compendium of Measures to Prevent Disease Associated with Animals in Public Settings, 2007," *Morbidity and Mortality Weekly Report* 56, no. RR05 (2007): 1–13, http://www.cdc.gov/mmwr/preview/mmwrhtml/rr5605a1.htm.

22. Jonathan S. Yoder and Michael J. Beach, "Cryptosporidiosis Surveillance—United States, 2003–2005," *Morbidity and Mortality Weekly Report* 56, no. SS05 (2007): 1–10, http://www.cdc.gov/mmwr/preview/mmwrhtml/ss5607a1.htm.

23. Edward Tyzzer, "A Sporozoan Found in the Peptic Glands of the Common Mouse," *Proceedings of the Society for Experimental Biology and Medicine* 5 (1907): 12–13.

24. Thomas H. Weller, *Ernest Edward Tyzzer: A Biographical Memoir* (Washington, DC: National Academy of Sciences, 1978).

25. G. Duffy, O. A. Lynch, and C. Cagney, "Tracking Emerging Zoonotic Pathogens From Farm to Fork," *Meat Science* 78 (2008): 34–42.

26. Sauonorine Tzipori and H. Ward, "Cryptosporidiosis: Biology, Pathogenesis and Disease," *Microbes and Infection* 4 (2002): 1047–58.

27. H. V. Smith et al., "Cryptosporidium and Giardia as Foodborne Zoonoses," *Veterinary Parasitology* 149 (2007): 29–40.

28. F. A. Nime et al., "Acute Entercolitis in a Human Being Infected with the Protozoan *Cryptosporidium*," *Gastroenterology* 70 (1976): 592–98; J. L. Meisle et al., "Overwhelming Watery Diarrhea Associated with *Cryptosporidium* in and Immunocompromised Patient," *Gastroenterology* 70 (1976): 1156–60.

29. H. Fujikawa et al., "Intestinal Cryptosporidiosis as an Initial Manifestation in a Previously Healthy Japanese Patient with AIDS," *Journal of Gastroenterology* 37 (2002): 840–43.

— 6 —
Ready-to-Eat?

When a food is "ready-to-eat" (RTE), it requires no additional cooking. Bagels, deli sandwiches, lunch meats, ice cream, produce, packaged potato salad and cole slaw, and cheeses are all examples of RTE foods. Most of us purchase these foods and eat them without thinking about the potential for getting sick. After all, isn't lunch meat cooked already? Cooking kills bacteria, so there is surely only minimal risk of getting sick from ingesting bacteria in precooked meats, right? Wrong. There are numerous microbiological pathogens that can contaminate food that is RTE. These include organisms that get into food during processing as well as those that contaminate food at the point of service.

Foods that are purchased to be eaten without additional cooking present a unique set of hazards to public health and for environmental health professionals to deal with. The final line of defense for most of us is cooking the product to kill pathogens, but this is not a food safety technique that can be readily monitored. The strategy that has been employed by environmental health professionals to strengthen the final line of defense has been extensive public education about food safety in the home. The government has supported educational campaigns, such as Fight BAC®, which is a consumer-oriented program designed to raise awareness about preventing bacteria from contaminating your food. While education programs are an important element of food safety, they generally focus on how consumers should cook their food or sanitize their kitchen. There is little information about preventing the spread of disease from foods that consumers will not cook or chill any further before eating—the RTE foods.

What information does exist about RTE foods may actually be confusing to consumers. For example, the brochure available from fightbac.org about handling fresh produce says, "Packaged fruits and vegetables labeled 'ready-to-eat,' 'washed,' or 'triple-washed' need not be washed." This advice from a prominent national food safety education program should probably be revised in light of recent outbreaks linked to bagged vegetables. It turns out that eating bagged salad without washing it first may not be such a good idea and may be a contributing factor in some of the outbreaks associated with fresh produce, including the 2006 spinach outbreak.

When a food is RTE, the manufacturer is not required to include any safe handling instructions on the packaging. This is according to the federal government, which defines the term "RTE" as follows:

A meat or poultry product that is in a form that is edible without additional preparation to achieve food safety, and may receive additional preparation for palatability or aesthetic, epicurean, gastronomic, or culinary purposes. RTE product is not required to bear a safe-handling instruction (as required for non-RTE products by 9 CFR 317.2(l) and 381.125(b)) or other labeling that directs that the product must be cooked or otherwise treated for safety, and can include frozen meat and poultry product.[1]

Because these products are not labeled with further cooking instructions, or even safe handling instructions, consumers might believe that they are always safe to eat as is. This can be a risky approach however as even highly processed foods, such as cooked sausages and deli meats, can harbor pathogens that can cause illness. It is for this reason that public health professionals and food safety experts are paying more attention to the ways in which microorganisms get into these foods and then spread throughout the food supply.

Viruses are arguably the most likely contaminants of RTE foods. This is because of their ability to effectively transmit from person to person and their heartiness in the environment. However, there are several bacteria that can cause severe disease and even death if they taint food that will be served without further cooking. These bacteria are especially problematic in food processing facilities that produce foodstuffs such as hot dogs, deli meats, and deli salads. This chapter focuses on several bacteria that can cause illness from foods that generally require minimal or no further cooking. Two of these pathogens, *Campylobacter* and *Listeria*, are important to health leaders in the United States as evidenced by the emphasis placed on them in national public health priorities.

HEALTHY PEOPLE EAT SAFE FOOD

Healthy People 2010 is a planning document containing public health objectives that were developed through collaboration among many governmental agencies. *Healthy People 2010* is actually an update of a document that was rolled out by the government 10 years earlier. *Healthy People 2000* was initiated by Julius Richmond, who was the Surgeon General of the United States from 1977 through 1981. The Surgeon General is the chief public health officer of the United States and this person reports directly to the Assistant Secretary for Health. One of the major roles of the Surgeon General is to educate the American public about health issues and the steps we can take to prevent disease. The Surgeon General warnings on tobacco products and alcohol are examples of ways the office gets health promotion messages to the public.

In 1979, the Office of the Surgeon General published a report, *Healthy People: The Surgeon General's Report on Health Promotion and Disease Prevention*, which laid the foundation for national objectives to improve public health in the United States.[2] This report emphasized the role that the public can play in preventing disease. One of the catalysts for this focus on prevention was the belief that people were becoming too reliant on medical care to maintain health. It is noted in this report that, although expenditures on health care were increasing, the statistics showed that Americans were not getting healthier. This is the basis for the argument that health promotion and prevention are critical elements in maintaining and improving the health of all people.

The 1979 report identifies the major risk factors to health as tobacco, alcohol and drug use, and injuries. Specific national health goals are also outlined in the document to improve the health of all population subgroups including infants, adolescents, and adults. These goals address environmental and behavioral factors that affect health as opposed to genetic factors that are not as easily controlled. The document also identifies some of the obstacles that stand in the way of health education and promotion designed to prevent disease. These obstacles include socioeconomic factors, personal attitudes, economic factors, and the state of our knowledge about health issues.

From the 1979 report, a nationwide initiative known as *Healthy People 2000* was developed. This initiative set goals for reducing disease from 22 priority areas including tobacco use, oral health, injury prevention, environmental health, and food safety. The food safety goals focused on reducing the disease burden from four specific pathogens that were considered the leading cause of illness at the time. These pathogens included

Campylobacter and *Listeria*, two bacteria that are commonly associated with RTE foods.

The Surgeon General made a commitment to update the *Healthy People* documents every 10 years. Part of the update includes an evaluation of the progress made toward achieving the objectives. The *Healthy People 2010* document is an update of *Healthy People 2000* and it sets additional objectives for food safety. The 2010 objectives recognize that progress was made in reducing the number of illnesses from the four specific pathogens, but that additional work is needed. The new report expands the objective of reducing their incidence even further, with the ambitious goal of cutting the incidence of disease from the major foodborne pathogens by 50 percent from the baseline year of 1997.

These objectives may be optimistic in that the resources needed to address public health in general and food safety in particular continue to compete with resources for other major programs such as defense, health care, and education. When it comes to *Campylobacter* and *Listeria*, even though there was some decline in the quantity of cases of illness from these pathogens from 1996 to 2001, there is current evidence to suggest that the gains made during this time may be reversing.[3] Since 2001, illness caused by *Campylobacter* has been rising and levels of *Listeria*-associated disease in 2006 were among the highest recorded since 2000.

THE MOST COMMON CAUSE OF DIARRHEA

Surveillance data indicates that the bacteria known as *Campylobacter jejuni* is one of the leading causes of diarrhea in humans. Since the levels of foodborne illness that we hear about in the news are only estimates based on reported incidence, it is likely that *Campylobacter* may actually be the number one reason why people get sick from food. It is the group of bacteria that are found most often in stool samples from people with diarrhea. The other bacteria that are contenders for the lead spot are all of the *Salmonella* species.

Even though *Campylobacter* are such important foodborne pathogens, they are not as well known as *Salmonella* or *E. coli*; this may be due to the fact that there have not been large-scale outbreaks connected to these bacteria. Rather, outbreaks tend to be smaller and more localized. These bacteria have been implicated as a major cause of outbreaks from drinking raw milk, something that is generally done at the local dairy and involves small numbers of people. Another reason why *Campylobacter* might not be as notorious as *Salmonella* has to do with the fact that these bacteria were not linked to human diarrhea until the 1980s, even though they may have been identified about 100 years before this association.

From Obscurity to Prominence

In 1886, Escherich, the scientist for whom *E. coli* is named, identified a spiral, rod–shaped bacteria in the stool of children with diarrhea. As with most of his work, he took detailed notes and published a paper in German describing the organism. However, according to historical accounts, the importance of his discovery was not noted until 100 years later at a conference in 1985.[4] In the intervening years between 1886 and 1985, veterinarians were recording the presence of these rod-shaped bacteria in sheep and cow feces.

The first time the bacteria were identified as a cause of human illness was in Illinois in 1938 when more than 350 inmates at a state prison became ill after drinking raw milk. The published account of this outbreak discusses the shape of bacteria as similar to what is known today as *Campylobacter*.[5] At this time in history however, *Campylobacter* were not categorized as a distinct bacteria; rather, they were grouped with other bacteria known as *Vibrio*.

From 1947 through the 1960s there were numerous accounts of human illness in which the spiral, rod-shaped bacteria were isolated from the blood of the victims. The breakthrough in identifying these bacteria as a major cause of human illness came in 1968 when researchers in Belgium were able to isolate the bacteria from the feces of a sick woman.[6] They described the bacteria as "spirally-shaped" and this shape distinguished these bacteria from the rest of the bacteria in the *Vibrio* classification. The Belgian researchers were instrumental in renaming and classifying these bacteria from *Vibrio* into the newly created *Campylobacter* genus, "campylo" meaning "curved."

Research related to *Campylobacter* has progressed rapidly since the 1960s, and in 1999 the bacteria became the first foodborne pathogen whose genome was sequenced. Genome sequencing allows scientists to understand the biology of an organism at a high level of detail by examining the patterns of DNA within the cells. It is a process that enhances the overall understanding of the organism in terms of its growth and its development.

Our enhanced understanding of *Campylobacter* may help minimize the spread of the pathogen. Genome sequencing of different *Campylobacter* species has taken place since the breakthrough in 1999 and all of this research is taking us near the point at which it won't be long until we will know more about *Campylobacter* than any other foodborne bacterial pathogen.

In general, genome sequencing work gives us a critical tool to accurately identify the species of the bacteria that are the most common cause of human illness.

The Jumping Bacteria

Unlike some of the other prominent bacteria, *Campylobacter* is not found in the environment; in fact, it is only found in warm-blooded animals. Therefore, when it contaminates the food or water supply, it does so by direct contact with feces of infected animals. One of the earliest documented outbreaks of illness from *Campylobacter* in the United States occurred in 1978 when about 2,000 people in Vermont were sick from drinking inadequately treated water. The water came from a source that was in an agricultural area and it is believed that the water became contaminated with livestock feces loaded with the bacteria. While infection with *Campylobacter* has been linked to public drinking water and several RTE foods and drinks, including bottled water and fresh vegetables, the most common sources of this pathogen are chicken and raw milk.[7]

Most of us are probably familiar with *Salmonella* as the pathogen that makes us sick from eating chicken or undercooked eggs. However, it may actually be *Campylobacter* that is the more likely cause of diarrhea associated with poultry products. Every time you purchase raw chicken, there is a high probability that you are getting campylobacter organisms for free. *Campylobacter* is found so often in the microbiological analysis of raw chicken that public health professionals recommend that consumers handle every package of chicken as if it were contaminated. This translates into special food safety procedures as chicken is prepared in the home or in restaurants.

When it comes to contracting campylobacteriosis from chicken, it is not eating raw or otherwise undercooked chicken that causes most problems. It is food preparation practices that create opportunities to spread disease. Any surface that comes in contact with contaminated raw chicken can become the vehicle for infecting what touches it next. This includes cutting boards, countertops, knives, and hands; herein is the real connection between *Campylobacter* and RTE foods. When a cutting board is used to cut chicken for sautéing and is then used to cut vegetables for a raw salad without being cleaned first, the bacteria can jump onto the carrots and celery to wait for the unsuspecting victim to take a bite.

This bacterial jumping is known as "cross-contamination" and is a major problem when it comes to spreading many disease pathogens, especially *Campylobacter*. Numerous studies have shown that the majority of chicken parts that are purchased at groceries are contaminated with *Campylobacter* and at least one study showed that the contamination is not as prevalent inside the meat as it is on the surface.[8] This suggests that the way in which these bacteria are most likely involved in cross-contaminating food is after the raw chicken is placed on the surface of a cutting board or counter. So, even without a lot of preparation work such as cutting or skinning involved, food contact surfaces can become ready harbors for the bacteria.

In order to minimize the risk of contaminating RTE foods with *Campylobacter*, some researchers are gathering data to help us understand the magnitude of cross-contamination under normal circumstances. Rather than contaminating chicken artificially under controlled circumstances such as laboratories, these researchers are using chicken that is naturally contaminated, and then examining bacterial levels in kitchens after food preparation. The results of this research suggest that *Campylobacter* is common on retail chicken parts and that these bacteria can cross-contaminate RTE foods to varying degrees. The extent of contamination depends in part on the type of contact surface, such as a wood versus a plastic cutting board. Furthermore, the type of chicken part involved seems to contribute to the intensity of the problem, with breasts suspected as a more effective transmitter of the pathogen than legs.[9] Since *Campylobacter* can be spread so efficiently from surfaces that they come in contact with, it is really up to consumers to minimize their risk for infection from these pathogens. Once again, it appears that the government's leading strategy for protecting American consumers from this pathogen has been to focus extensively on educating consumers about how to properly prepare meat, rather than enacting and enforcing regulations for industry.

Who's Minding the Chicken Store?

Remember that the consumer is the last line of defense against foodborne illness. With this in mind, relying on public education to prevent disease seems somewhat counter to the principles of public health protection. Public health practice is supposed to be the first line of defense against infectious disease. In adhering to this principle, wouldn't the government have to focus first and foremost on chicken producers and processors? What about the role they play in the spread of microbiological pathogens? The U.S. government has proven repeatedly that preventing contamination of our food supply is a task that they are unable to accomplish in an effective and consistent manner.

Perhaps one reason that the focus has shifted from regulating industry through inspections and regulations to educating the consumer is due to the explosion of the food industry itself. In 1995, the Food Safety Inspection

Service (FSIS) of the USDA proposed that all meat and poultry processors follow the lead of shellfish processors and incorporate the HACCP system to minimize the spread of pathogens. In the announcement of the proposed rule, FSIS explained that the meat and poultry processing industry had expanded too quickly for their inspectors to keep up with the oversight required by existing laws.[10]

One contributor to this problem was the automation of poultry and meat processing that sped up production lines. This automation and increased speed created an inability for inspectors to do an effective job in ensuring that the final product was not contaminated. FSIS said in their announcement that, "Automation has had a particularly great impact on poultry operations, where inspectors have had to face faster and faster line speeds, which today can be as high as 91 birds per minute."[11] At the time that the resources of FSIS were diminishing meat and poultry processing was gaining speed, leading to a strategy that addressed the problem by refocusing safety measures from industry to the consumer.

Since 1993, the chief public education approach to protect consumers from possible contamination in meat and poultry has been a mandatory label on all meat and poultry packaging at retail groceries that identifies "safe handling instructions." Included in the safe handling instructions is information on minimizing cross-contamination in the kitchen. Specifically, the text related to cross-contamination on meat and poultry packaging states: "Keep raw meat and poultry separate from other foods. Wash working surfaces (including cutting boards), utensils, and hands after touching raw meat or poultry."[12]

There is no way of knowing if this labeling has had any impact on reducing the incidence of campylobacteriosis; but it has cost plenty of money to implement. When they rolled out the labeling regulations, the USDA estimated that the mandatory safe handling label would cost industry and retailers between $76.1 and $92.1 million per year.[13] It is highly likely that most people do not even read the label, and if they do, it probably has very little impact on their food preparation techniques. In addition, mandatory food labeling may not be the best policy option in some cases, because the costs of implementing a new labeling system may far exceed the benefits of the label, especially if the label is never read. Furthermore, quantifying the costs and benefits is especially difficult in pure economic terms.[14]

There is no question that public education is an important component of improving food safety, but it cannot take place in a vacuum. This is especially true in the case of *Campylobacter*, as recent research suggests that it is possible to mass produce retail chicken that is free of the pathogen if the processing starts with uncontaminated chicken. Because *Campylobacter* does not survive for long periods in the environment, good sanitation on poultry farms and in food processing facilities can greatly reduce the risk.[15]

The *Campylobacter* Syndrome

The typical symptoms of campylobacteriosis begin a couple of days after exposure to the bacteria. These symptoms include a low-grade fever and diarrhea that can range from mild to bloody. Most healthy people will recover on their own in only a few days, but some cases may require treatment with antibiotics. This is especially the case if a victim is immunocompromised by age or a preexisting illness. What makes infection with *Campylobacter* different from infection with other common bacterial organisms, with the exception of *Salmonella*, is the risk of developing a chronic illness when these bacteria are ingested at high enough levels.

There have been several chronic illnesses linked to campylobacteriosis including arthritis. One of the emerging chronic disease issues is the relationship between campylobacteriosis and Guillain-Barré syndrome or GBS. Campylobacteriosis has been identified as the most common precursor to GBS and the *C. jejuni* is the species most commonly linked to GBS cases.[16]

GBS is a neurological condition that can lead to temporary paralysis. It is a rare disease but it can strike anyone regardless of age or health status. The syndrome starts when the immune system in the body attacks some of the peripheral nerves. For the victim, this can begin as just a tingling feeling in the arms and legs. However, the disease can progress to total paralysis and in a small number of cases the victim needs to be admitted to a hospital and placed on a mechanical ventilation unit in order to breathe. Patients who are admitted to intensive care units often suffer from additional conditions related to mechanical ventilation and many contract respiratory illnesses such as pneumonia.[17]

There is still research to be conducted to answer questions about the relationship between infection with *Campylobacter* and GBS. Nevertheless, the results to date are persuasive enough that many public health professionals agree that there is likely a connection. One of the most compelling stories about GBS can be found in the debate about what caused Franklin Delano Roosevelt to suffer from a condition that required the use of wheelchair for much of his adult life. Until recently, we were under the impression that FDR suffered an infection from the virus that causes polio. Now there is some evidence to suggest that the symptoms that FDR had were more likely to be caused by GBS than polio. This argument is all the more interesting because FDR's fight with what he thought was polio was a critical factor in the development of the polio vaccine.[18] If we had known then what we know now about *Campylobacter*, public health priorities may well have been different throughout much of the last century, and the health of Americans might be different today as well. Certainly there are no regrets about the advances made against polio, but one must now wonder if these advances were made on an incorrect assumption about the cause of FDR's health problems.

LISTERIA: THE "COOL" BACTERIA

While *Salmonella*, *E. coli*, and noroviruses are in the news almost daily, another serious pathogen is quietly spreading illness through foods that we grab on the run and eat without cooking. *Listeria* is a troubling group of bacteria because they do not follow the microbiological "rules" for growth. Whereas most bacteria thrive and grow at a neutral pH in a room-temperature environment, *Listeria* can grow at a lower pH and in colder temperatures. This means that some foods that we usually consider safe, such as lunch meats and sausages (because they are highly processed and precooked), may not be so safe after all, even if they are properly refrigerated.

The bacteria *Listeria* consists of six species: (1) *monocytogenes*; (2) *innocua*; (3) *seeligeri*; (4) *welshimeri*; (5) *ivanovii*; and (6) *grayi*. As with *Salmonella*, several of these species are further broken down by serovars. Of the six species, *monocytogenes* is the one of greatest concern to humans and it has been implicated most often in major foodborne outbreaks.

Royal Bacteria

In the arena of microbiology, *Listeria* is a relative newcomer. The bacteria was first identified and documented in 1924 by Everitt George Dunn Murray.[19] Murray was born in South Africa in 1890 and died in Canada in 1964. After his service during World War I, he became a leading researcher in England and is credited with identifying *Listeria* as a cause of meningitis during this time. Eventually he made his way to Canada and became the first chairman of the Department of Bacteriology at McGill University in 1931. During his tenure at McGill, Murray also assumed responsibility for coordinating the Canadian government's activities on biological warfare. He is said to have led a "secret" committee that coordinated testing to investigate the potential of biological organisms as weapons.[20]

Murray and his colleagues wrote about bacteria that were Gram-positive and rod-shaped that they discovered in laboratory rabbits in 1924. These bacteria were not previously described in published research; he called the new organism *Bacterium monocytogenes*.[21] It is generally accepted that the first time these bacteria were confirmed as a cause of human illness was in 1929 when Gram-positive, rod-shaped bacteria were identified in a German soldier. It took almost 60 years for food to be identified as the vehicle that spreads the bacteria in people.

As is the case with most microbiological discoveries, identifying the bacteria was paramount to understanding how it was spread in animals and people. The scientist credited with renaming this pathogen from *Bacterium monocytogenes* to *Listeria monocytogenes* was James Hunter Harvey Pirie. Pirie was an explorer and bacteriologist in the early 1900s and was a member of the Scottish National Antarctic Expedition from 1902 to 1904. In 1940 he published a letter in the journal *Nature* in which he proposed naming the bacteria *Listeria*, and apparently his proposal was accepted because the name was changed.[22]

Although *Listeria* were identified and renamed by the mid–twentieth century, it has been suggested that these bacteria played a major role in political upheaval in eighteenth-century England. It is possible that *Listeria* bacteria were the reason why Queen Anne was unable to produce an heir to the throne that she assumed in 1702, despite being pregnant at least 18 times.[23] Although there is some discrepancy in historical records, it is likely that that Queen Anne miscarried at least 12 times, bore two children who lived for less than a few hours after birth, had two children who lived for a year or less, and had one child who was stillborn. Her inability to produce an heir led to "political chaos" at the time and is one probable reason for the rise of the current parliamentary form of government in England.[24] Furthermore, because she left no heirs, the reign of King George ensued. If *Listeria* was the cause of the reproductive problems of Queen Anne, it may have ultimately contributed to the American Revolutionary War.

The most important research on *Listeria* began in the late 1940s when there was an outbreak of listeriosis in newborns and stillborns in Germany.[25] Bacteria consistent with the description of *Listeria* were found by a bacteriologist who was examining the blood and various organs of the infants, although he did not identify the bacteria as *Listeria* at the time. In the meantime another scientist was investigating a similar situation with infants at a different facility in Germany. This scientist, Heinz P. R. Seeliger, went on to collect almost 6,000 samples of the bacteria from all over the world.[26] Seeliger is also credited with writing the "bible" of *Listeria*, a book entitled *Listeriosis*, which was published in 1961.[27]

We now understand that *Listeria* species are ubiquitous in the environment. They have been found in water, soil, animal feed, and fecal matter at low levels.[28] We also understand the connection between listeriosis and spontaneous abortion and stillbirths, because the bacteria has the ability to pass through the placenta to newborns, an occurrence that can result in infant meningitis. It is not likely that we will ever be able to document that *Listeria* caused Queen Anne's inability to become a mother, but it is a plausible explanation.

With all of this history and the research regarding *Listeria* that was on-going throughout the early part of the twentieth century, it is somewhat surprising that these bacteria were not officially recognized as a significant cause of human foodborne illness until the 1980s.[29] Even more surprising is that there has actually been a great deal of research about *Listeria* completed in England and Wales, where there are more than 40 years of documented human health data related to *Listeria* food poisoning in these countries.[30]

The Magnitude of Listeria

One way to gauge the magnitude of *Listeria* contamination of RTE foods is by examining records of food recalls. In 2007, there were several recalls of RTE foods because of concerns over *Listeria* contamination, including one in Tennessee that involved more than 2,700 pounds of cooked, RTE chicken. This chicken was distributed to state correctional facilities and mental institutions. In June 2007, a New York food processor recalled about 140 pounds of chicken meals that were delivered to Stop & Shop grocery stores in New York and New Jersey. In May 2007, a California company recalled almost 7,000 pounds of turkey that was distributed in California, Colorado, Oregon, Texas, and Washington.

The largest recall in 2007 was by Carolina Culinary Foods when it re-called more than 2.8 million pounds of Oscar Mayer/Louis Rich chicken breast cuts and strips. These are the precooked strips that you can find in your grocery's meat section and many consumers put them on salads or sandwiches without further cooking. Carolina Culinary Foods produces the chicken products for Kraft foods and their tainted products were shipped nationwide. All told, *Listeria* was identified as the pathogen of concern in six of the approximately 40 food recalls in the United States in 2007.

When there is a recall because *Listeria* contamination is suspected, the federal government labels the recall as "Class I." This means that there is a reasonable chance that if someone consumes the infected product he or she will get sick. A Class I recall is the highest recall level because the human health risk is high in these instances. Although the recall process is explained in greater detail in Chapter 7, it is useful to remember that food recalls are voluntary, not mandatory, and that recalls address only a fraction of the actual problems with our food supply. In addition, a recall does not mean that someone has gotten sick from consuming the product; rather, it indicates that the pathogen was found either in the processing facility or in the product itself. One of the more common food products involved in *Listeria*-related recalls has been the ubiquitous hot dog.

Bacteria on a Bun

The federal government defines RTE foods as those that have been cooked according to food safety guidelines, including meat products, and need no further preparation before consumption. This would include hot dogs that are cooked and held at safe temperatures. There are numerous ways in which RTE foods can become contaminated with bacteria that cause foodborne illness. Let's examine the case of the hot dog as an example of how RTE foods may not actually be "ready to eat."

According to the National Hot Dog & Sausage Council, Americans spend almost 4 billion dollars every year on hot dogs and sausages. This expenditure amounts to about 1.5 billion pounds of these products bought at retail stores. Other interesting hot dog facts from the National Hot Dog & Sausage Council's Web site:

1. Americans will eat enough hot dogs at major league ballparks every year to stretch from RFK Stadium in Washington, DC, to AT&T Park in San Francisco.
2. New Yorkers consume more hot dogs than any other city—beating out Chicago and Los Angeles.
3. Chicago's O'Hare International Airport consumes six times more hot dogs— 725,000—than Los Angeles International Airport and New York's LaGuardia Airport combined.
4. On Independence Day, Americans will enjoy 150 million hot dogs—enough to stretch from DC to Los Angeles more than five times.
5. During "hot dog season"—Memorial Day to Labor Day—Americans typically consume 7 billion hot dogs—equivalent to 818 hot dogs consumed every second during that period.
6. U.S. soldiers in military posts around the world—from Fort Meyers in Arlington, VA, to Okinawa, Japan, to Aqaba, Jordon—consumed 2.4 million hot dogs last year.

The federal government does have standards related to hot dog production, but generally, hot dog manufacturers must comply with the same regulations as any other meat processing facility. The difference between hot dogs and some other meat products, a steak or roast for example, is that hot dogs are generally made by combining several meat products into one cylindrical delight. Many hot dogs contain more than just meat, they contain "by-products." According to the government, by-products can include hearts, livers, and kidneys. When there are by-products in hot dogs, they must be labeled as such.

Prior to the mad cow disease scare, mechanically separated beef could have been a component of your hot dog. When meat is mechanically separated from the bone, it is essentially forced through a sieve, bones and all, and comes out like a paste that is then formed into the tubular hot dog shape. Because of food safety concerns associated with the potential for bovine brain parts to end up in hot dogs, mechanically separated beef can no longer be used in American-made hot dogs. However, mechanically separated poultry can still be part of a hot dog sold in the United States.

The first place that hot dogs can become contaminated is at the processing facility through unsanitary practices pertaining to equipment and employees. Hot dogs are a highly processed food, meaning that many steps are required to create the final product. Each step in the process creates the potential for contamination. Once the hot dogs are finished and packaged, most are transported long distances to retail establishments. If there are any bacteria in the hot dog, they can reproduce to disease-causing levels if they are not kept under adequate refrigeration.

Once at the retail establishment, there are numerous ways in which the hot dog can become a further agent of disease. If the hot dog is cooked to the proper temperature (that is, 160 degrees Fahrenheit or higher), then it is likely that most bacteria will be killed. However, hot dogs are often held for long periods of time before serving. As a volunteer concessionaire at a Big Ten football stadium, I have been responsible for making hundreds of hot dogs at a single game and holding these hot dogs at high enough temperatures to ensure that sports fans will not get sick. This requires equipment that can hold the sandwiches at a temperature of at least 140 degrees Fahrenheit as verified with regular temperature checks.

Now ponder other places that hot dogs are purchased. Sidewalk vendors, convenience stores, gas stations, and school sports events. Considering the magnitude of our hot dog consumption, it is surprising that we don't get sick more often from eating them, or maybe we do but the incidence is unreported. Nevertheless, there are specific population groups that are warned not to eat hot dogs. For example, pregnant women should not eat hot dogs or lunch meat unless they are cooked to a high enough temperature to ensure that bacteria will be killed. This is a relatively new recommendation from the CDC based on their concern that *Listeria* can commonly contaminate these foods. One outbreak in 2002 that involved multiple states underscored the tragic consequences of fetal exposure to this bacterium. According to the CDC, during the 2002 outbreak, 46 cases were confirmed, seven people died, and there were three stillbirths or miscarriages. Turkey deli meat was identified as the way in which people were exposed to the pathogen and the meat was traced back to at least two processing facilities: Pilgrim's Pride Foods located in Franconia, Pennsylvania, and the Jack Lambersky Poultry Company, located in Camden, New Jersey.[31]

While there are still unanswered questions about the relationship between listeriosis and stillbirth, there is enough evidence to convince public health professionals that pregnant women should be very careful about their potential to be exposed to Listeria. If a pregnant woman is infected with the bacteria, she may just feel a little tired, or some minor stomach distress. These symptoms would probably not prompt the doctor to prescribe antibiotics. However, if not treated, the pathogen can pass through the placenta into the fetus resulting in an infection severe enough to cause miscarriage or stillbirth.[32]

The Dairy Bug

Many of the outbreaks of listeriosis are associated with dairy products, including cheeses and milk. The nature of Listeria, especially its ability to survive in refrigerated environments, creates a challenge to controlling it in food processing. Studies have documented the presence of the pathogen in all areas of food processing facilities, including floors, walls, drains, chillers, and employees.[33] These studies have taken place in numerous countries and in different types of plants, from dairy to meat-processing facilities.

One of the more common causes of illness is drinking unpasteurized milk and eating cheeses made from this milk. Two outbreaks in the United States in 2007 exemplify the risk of drinking raw milk. In December 2007, Massachusetts public health officials identified Listeria in raw milk as the most likely cause of two deaths in the summer of the same year. The victims were elderly men who had consumed the unpasteurized milk from a local dairy. During the same month down the coast in North Carolina, after identifying at least three cases of listeriosis, the North Carolina State Health Department warned the public, especially pregnant women, to not eat soft cheeses or drink raw milk.

A more serious incidence of listeriosis occurred in Massachusetts, also in 2007. The State Health Department confirmed that four cases of the disease were related to drinking pasteurized milk. This recent outbreak sets up a particularly threatening scenario involving some new strain of the bacteria that can survive pasteurization and thrive in commercialized dairy products. Because Listeria is such an important and deadly foodborne pathogen, it has caught the attention of U.S. politicians who may view its control as an opportunity to improve public health.

The Politics of Listeria

On May 6, 2000, President Bill Clinton announced a new initiative to reduce the number of foodborne illnesses and deaths caused by *Listeria* every year, specifically identifying RTE foods as a priority.[34] His initiative included requiring the USDA to develop regulations for the food industry to ensure that the risk of contamination with *Listeria* during processing is minimized and that foods remain safe during their entire shelf life. He also directed the USDA to develop a risk-based "action plan" that would identify the federal government's role in protecting the public from these bacteria. President Clinton gave the USDA 120 days to report back to him with their strategy for fulfilling his directive.

The politics of food safety emerged during the radio address in which Clinton announced his initiative. He argued that Congress was not cooperating to keep Americans safe from foodborne illness when he said: "Today, I call on the food industry to work with us as we develop our new *Listeria* strategy. And I call on Congress to help us strengthen food safety across the board. Just this week, unfortunately, the Congress took a major step backward by refusing to fully fund our food safety initiative. In fact, they've now voted to block funding for our new efforts to protect millions of American families from the dangers of *Salmonella* poisoning in eggs. We should be doing more, not less, to ensure the safety of our food."[35]

In response to the President's directive, the FDA drafted a risk assessment for *L. monocytogenes* in RTE foods.[36] Their risk assessment was completed and available for public comment in January 2001. After addressing the numerous comments they received, the FDA finalized the risk assessment in 2003.[37] As a result of their assessment of risk, the FDA noted that the risk of contracting illness from *Listeria* was the highest for those consuming hot dogs, deli meats, unpasteurized dairy products, and smoked seafood. The most dangerous foods in this group were identified as hot dogs, both unheated and reheated, and deli meats. Ultimately the FDA concluded that, although outbreaks are relatively rare, they can be very serious, especially to susceptible populations like pregnant women and the elderly.

The USDA recognizes the seriousness of *Listeria* and further evidence of this is found in a FSIS directive for inspections at facilities that process RTE foods.[38] This 2006 directive outlines specific steps that FSIS inspectors must take in order to minimize the risk of public exposure to this pathogen. Inspectors are provided with detailed directions describing how to inspect food contact and noncontact surfaces in processing facilities. In addition, a list of the most dangerous foods is provided. This list includes hot dogs, deli meats, deli salads, salt-cured products, and products labeled "keep frozen."

There has been no evaluation of the FDA's approach to minimizing *Listeria* exposure in RTE foods, but it is likely yet to come. Even if the government is ineffective at keeping our food safe, political maneuvers are one means of bringing the problems to light.

NOTES

1. Requirements of Special Classes of Product, *Code of Federal Regulations,* title 9, Sec. 430 (2007).

2. U.S. Department of Health Education and Welfare, *Healthy People: The Surgeon General's Report on Health Promotion and Disease Prevention* (Washington, DC: U.S. Government Printing Office, 1979), http://profiles.nlm.nih.gov/NN/B/B/G/K/_/nnbbgk.pdf.

3. CDC, "Preliminary FoodNet Data on the Incidence of Infection with Pathogens Transmitted Commonly through Food—10 States, 2006," *Morbidity and Mortality Weekly Report* 56, no. 14 (2007): 336–39.

4. J. P. Butzler, "*Campylobacter,* from Obscurity to Celebrity," *Clinical Microbiology & Infection* 10 (2004): 868–76.

5. A. J. Levy, "A Gastro-enteritis Outbreak Probably Due to a Bovine Strain of *Vibrio,*" *Journal of Infectious Diseases* 18 (1946): 243–58.

6. P. Dekeyser et al., "Acute Enteritis Due to Related *Vibrio*: First Positive Stool Cultures," *Journal of Infectious Diseases* 125 (1972): 390–92.

7. M. R. Evans, C. D. Ribeiro, and R. L. Salmon, "Hazards of Healthy Living: Bottled Water and Salad Vegetables as Risk Factors for *Campylobacter* Infection," *Emerging Infectious Diseases* 9, no. 10 (2003): 1219–25.

8. P. Luber and E. Bartelt, "Enumeration of *Campylobacter* spp. on the Surface and within Chicken Breast Fillets," *Journal of Applied Microbiology* 102 (2007): 313–18.

9. P. Luber et al., "Quantification of *Campylobacter* Species Cross-contamination During Handling of Contaminated Fresh Chicken Parts in Kitchens," *Applied and Environmental Microbiology* 72, no. 91 (2006): 66–70.

10. FSIS, "Pathogen Reduction; Hazard Analysis and Critical Control Point (HACCP) Systems; Proposed Rule," *Federal Register* 60, no. 23 (February 3, 1995), 6,773–889.

11. Ibid., 6776.

12. USDA, Safe Handling Label Text, http://www.fsis.usda.gov/News/Safe_Handling_Label_Text/index.asp.

13. Jordan C. T. Lin and Phil Kaufman, "Food Companies Offer View of Safe Handling Label For Meat and Poultry," *Food Review* (1995), http://findarticles.com/p/articles/mi_m3765/is_n3_v18/ai_18824581.

14. Eloise Golan et al., *Economics of Food Labeling* (2001), http://www.ers.usda.gov/publications/aer793/.

15. I. Cools et al., "Persistence of *Campylobacter jejuni* on Surfaces in a Processing Environment and on Cutting Boards," *Letters in Applied Microbiology* 40 (2006): 418–23.

16. S. Steve Yan et al., "*Campylobacter* Infection and Guillain-Barré Syndrome: Public Health Concerns from a Microbial Food Safety Perspective," *Clinical and Applied Immunology Reviews* 5 (2005): 285–305.

17. Rajat Dhar, Larry Stitt, and Angelika F. Hahn, "The Morbidity and Mortality of Patients with Guillain-Barré Syndrome Admitted to the Intensive Care Unit," *Journal of the Neurological Sciences* 264, no. 1/2 (2008): 121–28.

18. Costance Holden, "Did FDR Have Guillain-Barré?" *Science* 302, no. 5647 (2003): 981.

19. Jocelyn Rocourt, "The Genus *Listeria* and *Listeria monocytogenes*: Phylogenetic Position, Taxonomy, and Identification," in *Listeria, Listeriosis, and Food Safety*, 2nd ed., ed. Elliot T. Ryser and Elmer H. Marth (New York: Marcel Dekker, 1999), 1–20.

20. Donald H. Avery, *The Science of War: Canadian Scientists and Allied Military Technology During the Second World War* (Toronto: University of Toronto Press, 1998).

21. E.G.D. Murray, R. A. Webb, and H.B.R. Swann, "A Disease of Rabbits Characterized by a Hitherto Undescribed Bacillus *Bacterium monocytogenes* (n. sp.)," *Journal of Pathology and Bacteriology* 29 (1926): 407–39.

22. James Hunter Harvey Pirie, "*Listeria*: Change of Name for a Genus of Bacteria," *Nature* 145, no. 3668: 264.

23. W. B. Saxbe, Jr., "*Listeria monocytogenes* and Queen Anne," *Pediatrics* 49, no. 1 (1972): 97–101.

24. Ibid.

25. H. Hof, "History and Epidemiology of Listeriosis," *FEMS Immunology and Medical Microbiology* 35 (2003): 199–202.

26. Ibid.

27. Heinz P. R. Seeliger, *Listeriosis* (New York: Hafner, 1961).

28. David R. Fenlon, "Natural Environment," in *Listeria, Listeriosis, and Food Safety*, 21–38.

29. Elliot T. Ryser, " Foodborne Listeriosis," in *Listeria, Listeriosis, and Food Safety*, 299–358.

30. J. McLauchlin et al. "*Listeria monocytogenes* and Listeriosis: A Review of Hazard Characterization for Use in Microbiological Risk Assessment of Foods," *International Journal of Food Microbiology* 94 (2004): 15–33.

31. CDC, "Public Health Dispatch: Outbreak of Listeriosis—Northeastern United States, 2002," *Morbidity and Mortality Weekly Report* 51, no. 42 (2002): 950–51, http://www.cdc.gov/mmwr/preview/mmwrhtml/mm5142a3.htm; CDC, "Update: Listeriosis Outbreak Investigation," http://www.cdc.gov/od/oc/media/pressrel/r021104.htm.

32. Bala Swaminathan and Peter Gerner-Smidt, "The Epidemiology of Human Listeriosis," *Microbes and Infection* 9 (2007): 1236–43.

33. Robert Gravani, "Incidence and Control of Listeria in Food-Processing Facilities," in *Listeria, Listeriosis, and Food Safety*, 657–710.

34. White House, Office of the Press Secretary, "President Clinton Announces Aggressive Food Safety Strategy to Combat Listeria in Hot Dogs and Other Ready-To-Eat Foods" (May 6, 2000), http://www.foodsafety.gov/~dms/fs-wh20.html.

35. Clinton's radio address (May 6, 2000), http://www.clintonfoundation.org/legacy/050600-presidential-radio-address-on-food-safety.htm.

36. "Draft Assessment of the Relative Risk to Public Health from Foodborne *Listeria monocytogenes* among Selected Categories of Ready-to-Eat Foods" (2001), http://www.foodsafety.gov/~dms/mrisk.html.

37. FDA, *Quantitative Assessment of Relative Risk to Public Health from Foodborne Listeria monocytogenes Among Selected Categories of Ready-to-eat Foods* (2003), http://www.cfsan.fda.gov/~dms/lmr2-toc.html.

38. USDA, "Enforcement, Investigations, and Analysis Officer (EIAO) Assessment of Compliance with the Listeria Monocytogenes (Lm) Regulation and Introduction of Phase 2 of the Lm Risk-Based Verification Testing Program" (2006), http://www.fsis.usda.gov/OPPDE/rdad/FSISDirectives/10240.5.pdf.

— 7 —

Consumer Beware

In October 2007 a woman in Utah found a rat's head in a can of green beans. The spokesperson from the company that canned the product said, "there is no way that product could have hurt her. This rodent was rendered commercially sterile. We cook each can individually up to 265 degrees."[1] In other words, it was up to the woman who found the rat's head to decide whether she wanted to eat it or not—it was considered safe by the company. This reaction by the company sums up the food safety system in the United States—even though we have an extensive food safety system in place relative to other countries, when it comes right down to it, the ultimate burden is on the consumer to ensure that food is safe before it is eaten.

American consumers place a great deal of trust in the government to protect them from harmful contaminants in the food they eat. Why shouldn't they? When there is an outbreak, we often hear high-level governmental officials stating that our food supply is the "safest in the world." It may be the safest in the world, but recent widespread outbreaks of foodborne illness raise questions about our ability to keep it safe. There are several questions that are particularly difficult to answer, including "Is our food safe enough?" Who is ensuring that our food is as safe as it can be? How much responsibility and authority does the government have to protect consumers from unsafe food? Will we be able to ensure that our food supply is safe in the face of competition for finite resources?

Think about the numerous sources of our food, from fresh to packaged, from local to imported, and from homemade to retail. There is almost an unlimited number of ways that we can be exposed to unsafe food. Because this is an environmental health issue that affects everyone, the government places a high priority on ensuring that there are enough resources available for all of the food safety agencies—right? Well, not really. Government agencies responsible for protecting our food supply are underfunded, understaffed, and under the gun to keep up with all of the demands to ensure safe food.

The federal government is responsible for overseeing food manufacturing facilities, both those that provide fresh food and those that process food. It is also responsible for every step in the manufacturing process, from the farm to the retail establishment. The feds hand off the authority to state and local governments once food is either on the shelf for sale or on the menu for selection. Finally, the consumer is supposed to assume responsibility when he or she makes the purchase to take the food home for further preparation or to eat it in a restaurant. There are plenty of cases that show that consumers are often unwilling to assume this responsibility. Often when people get sick from eating something that was their choice, the result is not only a trip to the bathroom but a trip to a lawyer as well.

In addition to the government and consumers, another major element of the food safety system in the United States is the role of the food processor. These processors are regulated and inspected to the best of the government's ability considering the limited personnel and funding dedicated to this task. Due to the lack of resources, many facilities are not inspected as often as they should be. Even when they are, it is not possible for inspectors to watch the processing facility at all times. So, despite efforts on the part of government inspectors, sometimes unsanitary practices occur in the places that manufacture the food we eat. These practices can result in contaminated food that leads human disease or in unsavory, but not necessarily unhealthy, additives to food like a rat's head.

Once the contaminated food has left the facility, it will usually remain hidden unless somebody gets sick. Unfortunately the main alert system that we use to identify problems with the food industry is the occurrence of an outbreak; somebody has to get sick before we know there is a problem with the food. Although food processing facilities take many proactive steps to ensure safe food, sometimes the steps are reactionary and voluntary; the most obvious evidence of this comes in the form of the recall.

MANUFACTURES AND VOLUNTEERS

In 2007 there were unprecedented numbers of recalls of contaminated food products. There were also recalls of toys that were manufactured in China, a major pet food recall, and even a recall of Old Navy fleece jackets because the drawstring could pose a choking hazard. According to Recalls. gov, there were 51 recalls of consumer products in November 2007 alone. There are several governmental agencies and commissions responsible for overseeing the recall system for consumer products, automobiles, and food. However, the agencies have varying levels of authority when it comes to requiring a recall.

Consumer product recalls are coordinated by the Consumer Product Safety Commission (CPSC). The CPSC is an independent agency that is not part of any federal department; it is run by three commissioners and a staff of about 420 people who are responsible for ensuring that the American public is safe from more than 15,000 product lines. The CPSC has authority to order recalls of consumer products if the product violates safety standards. There does not have to be any evidence that someone has actually been injured or sickened by the product. The 2007 recalls that involved toys containing lead paint is one example of a major recall of millions of pieces initiated because the items violated standards for lead—not because anyone was actually harmed by the products.

Vehicle recalls in the United States are handled by the National Highway Traffic Safety Administration (NHTSA). Although automobile manufactures often voluntarily recall cars because of defects, the NHTSA is authorized to order recalls of vehicles if it is determined that the vehicle contains defects that could seriously harm consumers. Examples of these defects include poor tires, steering component problems, and airbag malfunctions. As with the consumer product recalls, there is usually not evidence that someone has been harmed by the problem; rather the recall is purely precautionary.

Recalls of food, drugs, and cosmetics are handled somewhat differently than consumer products or vehicles. Two government agencies are involved in recalls of these consumables, the FDA and the FSIS. The FDA is part of the Department of Health and Human Services (DHHS) and the FSIS is in the Department of Agriculture. So, coordination issues should be immediately apparent in the case of food recalls.

Another major difference between food product recalls and consumer product and vehicle recalls is that food recalls are totally voluntary. Neither the FDA nor the FSIS has the authority to order any food manufacturer to recall product. A company may choose to recall a product voluntarily, which suggests that food recalls often do not take place until there is evidence that someone has actually been harmed by the product. For example, on September 29, 2007, a major food manufacturer issued a recall of more than 21 million pounds of ground beef because 25 people were confirmed ill after ingesting *E. coli* bacteria. If there was no reported illness, the recall would not have taken place, and the contaminated beef could remain in the food supply. This recall is one of more than 40 that the FSIS listed in 2007.

While some consumers may feel reassured that a recall minimizes their risk of exposure to contaminants in food, keep thinking about the fact that food recalls are a voluntary activity. Food manufacturers voluntarily pull products off the market and alert consumers to potential problems with the food. Most Americans are probably unaware that the government does not require companies to recall unsafe food products. A food recall is not an enforcement action and the federal government (i.e., the FDA) can only recommend that a company recalls suspicious foods.

Recalls managed by the FDA and FSIS are divided into three classes based on the potential for the contaminated food to cause imminent health threats. A Class I recall is the most serious and suggests that the food has a high probability of causing serious health problems or even death. For example, if *Listeria* bacteria are identified as a cause of illness and linked to a specific food, this could result in a Class I recall. A Class II recall is less serious and any health effects that may occur from exposure are considered reversible. The Class III recall is the least serious and occurs when there is not likely to be any adverse health effects, even if people are exposed. Most of the pathogens discussed in this book would lead to a Class I recall if they are suspected in foods. An example of a Class I recall occurred in summer 2007 when one of the most potent microbiological agents was discovered in canned food.

"These Products Can Hurt People"

A recent Class I recall involved the case of potential contamination of canned chili sauces and other chili products in 2007. There are normally about 25 cases of botulism in the United States in any given year and, according to the CDC, almost all of these cases are caused by consuming foods that were canned in the home. Since the bacteria lives in soil, if an inexperienced home canner does not wash the product or sterilize the jars adequately, the toxin can reproduce while the jars are being stored. In the summer of 2007, the CDC became aware of four cases of botulism, two in Texas and two in Indiana.[2] The CDC was also investigating a suspicious case of botulism in California. It was unusual to see four simultaneous cases of this illness in different states, especially states that are so far apart in proximity. If this situation was caused by home canning, then it would imply that the victims had some type of relationship that enabled them to obtain the contaminated product from a common source.

The Texas cases involved two siblings, and a married couple in Indiana was the second set of cases. There was no relationship found among the cases, so environmental health officials suspected that this might be an outbreak linked to a product that was commercially processed, rather than inexperienced home canning. If this was true, it would be the first time there was a recorded outbreak of botulism from commercially canned food in more than 30 years.[3] Furthermore, if this was a nationwide outbreak, it was a critical situation because it involved the microbiological pathogen that produces the most deadly toxin known to humankind. A small dose of the bacteria, *Clostridium botulinum*, can rapidly produce a toxin that paralyzes bodily functions leading to death.

C. botulinum is a member of a group of bacteria that forms spores. These spores are surrounded by a hard shell, making them resistant to many of the standard control techniques. These bacteria are unique in more ways than just their ability to produce spores. When applying FATTOM principles for food safety as discussed in Chapter 1 of this book, one of the factors is the availability of oxygen. Most bacteria need some oxygen to grow, but *C. botulinum* is an anaerobe, meaning that it reproduces best in an environment depleted of oxygen—they love canned food.

I recall grocery shopping with my mother at a young age. Whenever we got to the canned food isle, she would always take great care to examine all of the cans she put into the cart. No bulging or even dented cans ever made it into our grocery bags. At the time, I remember being quite annoyed and embarrassed that she would look the cans over so carefully. I also thought that this was just another example of her obsessive orderliness. Now I understand that she was actually looking for signs of botulism in the canned food. If the bacteria were reproducing inside, the can could bulge as the bacteria competed for space with the chicken noodle soup or green beans.

My grandparents did a lot more home canning than we do now, so my mother understood at a young age the importance of scrutinizing commercially canned food. Botulism is one of the most important reasons why it is so critical to perform meticulous sterilization while home canning. If any of these bacteria should happen to be on the jar or in the product being canned, sealing the jar creates a virtual utopia for their growth. Students in my college classes today do not even know that it is possible to can your own fruits and vegetables, let alone have an understanding of the importance of looking for signs of botulism in the cans they purchase at the grocery store. Clearly, we are fortunate that botulism in commercially canned foods is a rarity.

The cases in July 2007 were eventually linked to commercially processed chili sauce and the company that produced the sauce voluntarily recalled the product. The chili sauce recall involved canned foods from Castleberry's Food Company in Augusta, Georgia. This company was founded in the early 1920s in Augusta, Georgia and remained a family-run company until 2004. Connors Bros. Income Fund, which is Canada's largest consumer products income fund, acquired Castleberry's by merging its subsidiary Bumble Bee, headquartered in San Diego, with the Georgia-based company. This merger created one of the largest canned meat processors in the United States. Connors Bros. already was the largest canned seafood company prior to the merger.

Castleberry's first notified the public of its voluntary recall on July 18, 2007, and identified 10 specific products that were suspected to be the source of the outbreak. All of the products were canned chili products. On July 21, 2007, the company expanded the recall to include more than eighty types of canned chili products and four types of canned dog food. Remember that food recalls do not usually occur until illness has already been documented, and this was the case with the botulism recall. At least four people were seriously ill before the recall began.

The chili recalled that could contain botulism bacteria was so deadly that the CDC recommended that consumers dispose of their suspicious canned products by double-bagging the unopened cans in plastic bags and putting them in trash receptacles that are not inside the house. This exceptional recommendation was made just in case the cans were to rupture during disposal, so that the plastic bags would catch the contents and bacteria would not be released into the environment.

In the midst of a recall, good communication is essential. The media has a critical role to play, because in most cases, a recall requires consumers to take immediate action. This is especially challenging during nationwide or widespread recalls. How can you effectively let everyone in the country know that there might be a ticking time bomb in their cupboard? During a conference call with the media on July 24, 2007, Captain David Elder, a public health officer in the FDA's Office of Enforcement, summed up both the urgency and the frustration of using the recall system to protect public health when he said, "These products can hurt people and have to be off the store shelves, and consumers have to discard any that they have at home."[4]

According to the Connors Bros. quarterly report ending in September 2007, the recall cost the company more than $15 million, which was actually good news. When the recall began in July, they estimated that it would cost at least twice that amount, more than $35 million. The estimate included allowances for customer returns and the estimated financial impact that the recall would have on their brand name. In addition, the Augusta, Georgia, facility was closed for more than two months during the recall, leading to an additional economic effect on the company's inventory. Insurance covered some of the recall expenses; however, the company underestimated the re-sources needed to recall and destroy the recalled product. On the other hand, they had overestimated the funds that would be needed to process customer product returns.

The overestimation of cost of customer refunds is another indicator of the difficulty in recalling processed foods during a multistate outbreak. Consumers have to be informed about the danger and given instructions to return the product. In this case, the CDC was advising people to carefully and immediately dispose of the products, while the company was allowing consumers to return the product. Consumers could choose to throw their products away or get a refund, but not both—apparently most people threw their chili sauce away because Connors Bros. did not spend nearly as much as they thought they would for refunds.

One additional factor that makes processed foods especially difficult to manage in a recall situation is their long shelf lives. This means that someone could easily eat canned chili that was processed more than one year earlier. During the year that the chili sauce sat in someone's cupboard, the process-ing facility continued to produce the food, so tracing the source of a patho-gen is almost impossible. In the case of the 2007 botulism recall, products that were processed over a two-year period were involved, a situation that could have involved billions of cans.

The greatest unknown expense in this type of recall situation is often the company's legal expenses should litigation ensue. In any event, the financial loss to Connors Bros. as of November 2007 was at least $15 million. The costs were borne by the company as a result of the illness of four, perhaps five people who all eventually recovered from the disease. Legal expenses related to this case may be yet to come. When a company issues a recall, it probably appears as an admission of guilt to many. The fact that recalls are voluntary does not matter to people who have suffered from contaminated food.

The U.S. government has less authority to take cans contaminated with botulism off store shelves than it does to remove a sweatshirt with a poten-tially unsafe drawstring. How did we get to this place in time when we rely on the voluntary activities and good will of food manufacturers to protect us against imminent health threats? All we need to do is look at resource al-location for food safety activities in the United States and we get a sense of some of the major problems that might help provide an answer.

"ONE OF THE SAFEST FOOD SUPPLIES IN THE WORLD?"

The first federal food safety law was passed in 1906, largely in response to public outcry over the conditions described by Upton Sinclair in his book *The*

Jungle. Although a work of fiction, the descriptions of the stockyards and the meatpacking industry in the book alarmed the public and led to pressure on the government to do something about it. More than 100 years later there are still problems with the food supply, although they are not as blatant as those laid out in *The Jungle.* One of the biggest problems in managing food safety is that jurisdiction cuts across several agencies at all levels of government.

Entire books can be written on the subject of the food safety system in the United States; it is that complicated. Ensuring safe food involves a complex collaboration among all levels of government, food manufacturers and processors, farmers, and consumers. Legislators attempt to manage the system through laws, regulations, and policy, which gives the illusion of a coordinated approach. For example, the FDA and USDA are responsible for ensuring safe poultry and meat, the EPA is responsible for regulating pesticides on food, and local health departments take over when it comes to retail food service.

Mike Leavitt, the Secretary of the DHHS, said at a Congressional hearing in December 2007, "Americans enjoy one of the safest food supplies in the world." This is a true statement that is commonly uttered by officials at all levels of government, especially in the middle of a nationwide outbreak. The problem with the assurance is that with each new outbreak or recall, consumers are becoming less inclined to be reassured.

Food safety is an illusion because of the nature of our food supply and the lack of resources available to protect it. When the meat in a single hamburger patty comes from 10 different farms, the risk of eating a contaminated sandwich increases. When the spinach in a bag of RTE salad is shipped from California to New Jersey, the probability of eating an unsafe salad becomes greater than if the spinach was bought from a local farmer. When the local health department has one environmental health professional to inspect six hundred restaurants per year, there is a reason to be concerned about the safety of your food. By the time food is put on your plate it may have been inspected by several agencies or none—the latter is becoming the norm.

There are two major federal government departments and one federal agency that work to ensure food safety. The DHHS and the USDA are members of the president's cabinet and several agencies within these departments are involved with food safety. The EPA is not a cabinet-level agency, but it is involved in protecting the food supply.

Department of Health and Human Services (DHHS)

Within the DHHS there are several agencies with food safety responsibilities including the FDA and the CDC. The FDA is the lead agency responsible for ensuring that domestic food and cosmetics are safe. The administrator of the FDA is the commissioner, and within the FDA there are six centers and an Office of Regulatory Affairs. While a major function of the FDA is regulating and ensuring the safety of drugs, the agency also has food safety tasks. The Center for Food Safety and Applied Nutrition (CFSAN) and the Center for Veterinary Medicine (CVM) are the two centers in the FDA that are in charge of food safety.

The statement from the head of the DHHS that America's food supply is the safest in the world is problematic especially considering that the advisory committee to his chief agency responsible for food safety within the DHHS says "the nation's food supply is at risk" and "our food supply grows riskier every year."[5] In November 2007, a subcommittee of the FDA Science Board Advisory Committee, which advises the FDA commissioner about science and technology issues, published a scathing report about conditions at the FDA.

After a year-long investigation, the subcommittee concluded that the FDA is in a state of crisis. In the report, words like "dangerous," "peril," and "badly crippled" are used to describe the current state of affairs at the FDA. The crisis is based on 20 years of underfunding, a lack of trained staff, and an information technology system that is "problematic at best—and at worst it is dangerous." The problems cited in the report involved the two centers in the FDA that are the front line protectors of the nation's food supply.

The CFSAN is the center within the FDA that is charged with protecting public health from potential hazards in the domestic and imported food supply. The priorities of CFSAN include food defense, food safety, nutrition and labeling, dietary supplements, and cosmetics. The CFSAN is the primary food safety regulatory and consumer education arm of the FDA. It is involved in regulating food additives; investigating biotechnology; conducting research; labeling food products; overseeing dietary supplements; monitoring foods once they are on the market; educating consumers and the food industry; and cooperating with state, local, and international governments.[6]

The CVM oversees food-producing animals, and their work includes regulating the use of antibiotics and other animal feed additives. The CVM was the central government entity involved with the nationwide pet food recall in 2007. The CVM was alerted to the problem with pet food when the manufacturer contacted them to report that 14 animals had died. Five of these were reported by owners and the other nine died while the pet food manufacturer was testing the product at their processing facility. During this recall, the CVM collected samples, conducted additional inspections, handled the press, and answered questions from concerned pet owners. The CVM also worked with the USDA when it was discovered that animals for human consumption also had ingested tainted feed.

The subcommittee that completed the review of the FDA in 2007 noted that the CFSAN and CVM are the centers in the agency that face the most series deficiencies in their ability to accomplish their missions. The food safety approach employed in these two centers is one of "management by crisis," which has contributed to high rates of staff turnover and an inadequately prepared workforce in general. This management approach has also limited the centers' ability to use sound science in making decisions, a problem that could lead to approvals of substances that might be a threat to public health. The activities of the FDA in general and the CFSAN in particular are continuing to evolve away from strictly enforcement and inspections and towards product review. An example of a food product review took place in the mid-1990s when the agency approved Olestra as a fat substitute.

Overall, the FDA has a tremendous amount of responsibility when it comes to food safety, including inspecting food processing facilities and warehouses; testing food additives and preservatives; coordinating recalls; educating consumers; and developing food safety guidance documents. The FDA is also responsible for regulating the multibillion-dollar bottled water industry. Once water is bottled, it is considered a food by the federal government and is regulated as such. Bottled water is a major industry in the United States, and its per capita consumption has more than doubled since 1993.[7] The responsibilities of the FDA continue to expand with each additional food processing plant, and the increasing demand for imported foods. While their tasks are increasing, their resources are not.

As we have seen an increase in foodborne outbreaks, we have also seen a reduction in the food safety workforce at the FDA. In 1988, the FDA had 7,039 full-time employee equivalents or FTEs. In 2007, the number of FTEs at the FDA had risen to 7,856. However, with respect to food safety programs, 3,082 FTEs were identified as food safety staff in 2004. By 2008, this level had dropped to 2,702, a loss of about 10 percent of the workforce.[8] The effect of the shrinking resource base has contributed to an "appallingly low inspection rate" and a finding that the agency's food safety mission has been "severely eroded."[9]

At a time when keeping our food safe is becoming more complicated and important, one of the main agencies responsible for protecting public health is suffering from a lack of resources. As of early 2008, a workforce of a little more than 2,700 FTEs is responsible for ensuring that all food that is processed or imported into the United States and sold in more than 300,000 food establishments will not make us sick.

President Bush recognized that there is problem with ensuring food safety, especially in that of imported products. Evidence of this understanding can be found in his Executive Order (EO) signed in July 2007. This EO established an Interagency Working Group on Import Safety. The mission of the group is "to identify actions and appropriate steps that can be pursued, within existing resources, to promote the safety of imported products."[10] Essentially this group, which is chaired by the Secretary of the DHHS (or designee), will be reviewing existing procedures related to the safety of imported products and making recommendations for changes. While this sounds like priorities may be strengthening toward enhancing food safety programs, there is a catch—the changes that are recommended are not to require additional resources. The lack of new resources implies that, if re-prioritization needs to take place, then some other program will suffer the consequences of a reduction of resources, setting up a "robbing Peter to pay Paul" scenario.

It should be clear that the underlying cause of the problem at the FDA is the lack of connection between those who mandate growth in agency responsibilities and those who decide how the budget will be allocated. The subcommittee that authored the 2007 report noted that from 1987 to 2007, Congress enacted 125 new statutes that required action on the part of the FDA and not a single statute was accompanied by additional resources. In thinking about the impact of these unfunded mandates, one can't help but imagine a scene of chaos at the agency. Staff that is already stretched as tightly as it can go tries to keep up with current workloads, while new mandates and responsibilities are dumped on them on a regular basis. The fascinating outcome of this process is a Congress that is angered and surprised by the inability of the FDA to adequately protect public health.

Another agency within the DHHS that is heavily involved in food safety is the CDC. Within the CDC, there are centers, divisions, and branches. The National Center for Zoonotic, Vector-borne, and Enteric Diseases (NCZVED) takes the lead on food safety. Each center in the CDC is made up of divisions, and the Division of Foodborne, Bacterial, and Mycotic Diseases inside of the NCZVED is the primary division behind food safety initiatives. Finally, there are several branches within the division that share the lead on food safety.

Unlike the FDA and its centers, the centers in the CDC have no regulatory authority. The CDC is principally a scientific research organization that provides pathogen detection, epidemiology studies, and surveillance. The branches in the NCZVED include an enteric diseases epidemiology branch and an enteric diseases laboratory branch. These branches focus on finding the causes of human enteric illness and provide recommendations for preventing further illness.

One of the most important roles that the CDC plays is in its surveillance of foodborne illness. There are three initiatives that are critical for quickly identifying outbreaks and their possible causes: FoodNet, PulseNet, and the National Antimicrobial Resistance Monitoring System (NARMS). FoodNet is the surveillance initiative that consists of 10 sites around the country that are actively monitored by the CDC. This means that CDC staff contact the laboratories that serve the 10 sites to gather data about confirmed cases of nine specific foodborne pathogens.

According to the CDC, the 10 sites in FoodNet represent about 44.9 million people, or about 15 percent of the U.S. population. The data collected at the FoodNet sites are used to indicate what types of foodborne illness trends may be occurring in the country. The most recent report about disease incidence at FoodNet sites indicates that cases of *Campylobacter* and *Listeria* have declined since 1996; however, cases of *E. coli* O157:H7, *Salmonella*, and *Vibrio* have increased.[11]

PulseNet is a nationwide network of laboratories that conduct DNA analysis of pathogens. The purpose of this type of analysis is to help identify common strains of microbiological organisms and to link cases of illness that may be occurring in different parts of the country. NARMS consists of laboratories at several agencies that analyze samples to look for changes in common microbiological pathogens, and their ability to resist antibiotics. Since 1996, NARMS has provided valuable information about foodborne pathogens, and this information is being used in other countries as well as the United States.

Unlike the FDA, there has been no recent scathing report about the inadequacies at the CDC, and public opinion polling has historically given the CDC high rankings relative to other government agencies.[12] The budget for food safety activities within the CDC has remained flat since 2006. There has been no change in the $28 million figure that was allocated to the food safety branches since 2006; furthermore, the budget request for 2008 was exactly the same as the 2006 allocation.

It is worth noting that the budget for food safety activities at the CDC in 2004 was over $36 million. So, in four years, there has been an $8 million or 22 percent reduction in food safety funding within the CDC. Some of this difference can be attributed to reorganization of agency activities, while some if it is also attributed to their growing focus on global disease detection, such as a shift to prioritizing pandemic flu activities and addressing homeland security issues.

Department of Agriculture

The USDA collaborates with the FDA and the CDC in many food safety initiatives including FoodNet and NARMS. However, this department has a major regulatory role in protecting the nation's food supply. The FSIS is housed in the USDA. According to their Web site, FSIS is "the public health" agency inside the USDA and their major responsibilities include ensuring the safety of meat, poultry, and egg products.

FSIS operates under three major federal laws that require mandatory inspections of all facilities that process meat, poultry, and egg products. There are 7,865 meat, poultry, and egg inspectors affiliated with FSIS. In addition to federal inspectors, there is a network of state inspectors that focus on slaughtering facilities. The career path for a food inspector at the FSIS begins in a slaughterhouse, where responsibilities include examining animals before and after slaughter. After spending time in a slaughterhouse, it is possible to be promoted to inspecting a food processing facility and testing for microbiological contaminants of food products. FSIS is in charge of inspecting more than 250,000 products that include meat, poultry, and egg products. The magnitude of the products under the authority of the FSIS means that not all products can be tested for pathogens.

A pivotal moment in the history of the FSIS came in 1993 with the *E. coli* O157:H7 outbreak in the Pacific Northwest. The result of this outbreak was public demand that the government do more to ensure that ground meat products were as safe as possible. These demands led to new science-based food safety management systems, and the FSIS was responsible for issuing the federal regulation requiring meat and poultry processors to use HACCP methods. As discussed previously, HACCP is a comprehensive planning process that addresses critical steps in the food production process and methods to use if there are any problems with the steps.

In addition to inspecting facilities, FSIS is responsible for coordinating recalls. The primary goal of FSIS is to ensure that the public is informed about recalled food products. They do this through the use of the Internet and with press releases. The FSIS may issue a request to a food processor for a recall if their staff has tested food products and found evidence that the food is contaminated. There may be cases in which FSIS inspectors recommend a recall due to unsanitary conditions at a processing facility. Sometimes the processor finds a possible contamination source in the facility and lets the FSIS know that there is a potential problem.

The 2008 budget for the FSIS includes an unprecedented $1.1 billion request. Most of the budget for FSIS covers the cost of inspections of the 6,282 establishments and 121 import stations that are its responsibility.[13] In addition to the federal inspectors, there are inspectors at the state level and most of these are individuals responsible for slaughterhouses. Even though inspectors are supposed to be on-site at all slaughterhouses, the largest beef recall in U.S. history occurred in February 2008 from a facility that was complying with federal regulations.

The Humane Society of America released video footage of cattle too sick to walk on their own being forced into the meat supply at a Westland/Hallmark meat company in California, where there were USDA inspectors on site. These so-called downer cows are of concern due to the potential for mad cow disease. The result of the release of the video was a recall of more than 143 million pounds of ground meat. A large percentage of this ground meat was either already eaten, being prepared, or on its way to numerous schools throughout the country. In late February at least two inspectors who were in charge of overseeing the plant were suspended from their jobs—on paid administrative leave.

State and Local Governments

The federal government does not conduct routine inspections of retail food establishments; this is a job left up to state and local governments. In 1973, the field staff at the FDA conducted 34,919 inspections of domestic and foreign food establishments, while in 2006 the field staff conducted just 7,783. The reduction in federal field staff and the overall condition of food safety programs at the federal level has led to increased reliance on local governments to protect consumers across the country.

The local government agencies that shoulder most of the responsibility for food safety are local health departments either at the county or city level. In order to explain how the division of labor works, let's take a look at the state of Ohio as an example. In Ohio there are 87 counties, but 132 health districts. Some of the districts have jurisdiction only over cities. For example, in Cuyahoga County, there is county health department, but it does not cover the city of Cleveland, which has its own health department. Smaller, rural counties may only have one health department for the entire county, but the urban counties that house Columbus, Cleveland, Toledo, Akron, Cincinnati, and Dayton have more than one health department.

The local health departments have environmental health staff sanitarians that have the principle responsibility for food safety. Some of the health departments have several sanitarians, while other departments may only have one assigned to inspect all of the retail food establishments. This approach, which is common in most of the states, means that food safety is inconsistent throughout the state. Environmental health personnel are typically responsible for more than just food safety, so it is not uncommon for there to be extended periods of time between inspections at some facilities.

Even under the best budgetary conditions, local health departments suffer from severe resource shortages. These departments are in districts that are funded in large part by taxes from residents in the service area. As the tax burden increases, in addition to all of the other economic woes that the country is facing, the belt at local health departments is sure to get tighter and tighter. The implication of this approach to food safety at the point of sale is that it is truly not possible for resource-depleted local health departments to comprehensively oversee the distribution of safe food to consumers across the country.

NOTES

1. *Columbus Dispatch*, October 8, 2007.

2. CDC, "Botulism Associated with Commercially Canned Chili Sauce—Texas and Indiana, July 2007," *Morbidity and Mortality Weekly Reports* 56, no. 30 (2007): 467–69, http://www.cdc.gov/mmwr/preview/mmwrhtml/mm5630a4.htm.

3. Ibid.

4. FDA Press Conference on Chili Products (Botulism) Recall, July 24, 2007, http://www.fda.gov/bbs/transcripts/transcript072407.pdf.

5. U.S. House of Representatives, Subcommittee on Science and Technology, *FDA Science and Mission at Risk* (December 3, 2007), http://www.fda.gov/ohrms/dockets/ac/07/briefing/2007-4329b_02_00_index.html.

6. CFSAN, *Overview* (2001), http://www.cfsan.fda.gov/~lrd/cfsan4.html.

7. Beverage Marketing Corporation, *The 2004 Beverage Marketing Directory, Twenty-Sixth Edition* (New York: Beverage Marketing Corporation, 2004).

8. CFSAN, *CFSAN Budget Narrative* (2008), http://www.fda.gov/oc/oms/ofm/budget/2008/1-BudgetNarrativeCFSAN.pdf.

9. Subcommittee on Science and Technology, *FDA Science and Mission at Risk*.

10. George W. Bush, *Executive Order Creating Interagency Working Group on Import Safety* (2007), http://www.whitehouse.gov/news/releases/2007/07/20070718-4.html.

11. CDC, "Preliminary FoodNet Data on the Incidence of Infection with Pathogens Transmitted Commonly through Food—10 States, 2006," *Morbidity and Mortality Weekly Report* 56, no. 14: 336–39, http://www.cdc.gov/mmwr/preview/mmwrhtml/mm5614a4.htm?s_cid=mm5614a4_e.

12. The Harris Poll, *CDC, FAA, NIH, FDA and FBI Get Highest Ratings of Eleven Federal Governing Agencies* (2004), http://www.harrisinteractive.com/harris_poll/index.asp?PID=524.

13. USDA, *FY 2008 Budget Summary and Annual Performance Plan*, http://www.obpa.usda.gov/budsum/fy08budsum.pdf (accessed January 15, 2008).

— 8 —

Unusual Priorities: From Bad Apples to Mad Cows

On April 15, 1996, the topic on the *Oprah Winfrey Show* was food safety; however the edited version of the show ultimately focused only on the issue of mad cow disease. The panel on the show consisted of: Howard Lyman, executive director of the Humane Society's *Eating With Conscience*; Gary Weber, a representative from the National Cattlemen's Beef Association; and Dr. Will Hueston from the USDA. In the course of the discussion Howard Lyman explained that mad cow disease is thought to be the result of feeding sick cows to well cows, a practice that is essentially cannibalism. This prompted Oprah to say, "It has just stopped me cold from eating another burger!"[1]

This 10-word sentence uttered by one of the most influential people in the United States led to a public outcry about how we feed cattle, a new focus on intensive agriculture, congressional involvement, and a high-profile lawsuit filed on behalf of the beef industry, naming Oprah as the defendant. After the show, the demand for beef plummeted and the cattle industry sued Oprah for causing what they estimated was more than $10 million in damage to their industry. The notable aspect of the lawsuit was that the Texas Cattlemen's Association brought the suit under a law that was specifically designed to protect the agriculture industry from bad press, a law that started with apples.

THE FORBIDDEN FRUIT

Apples are the all-American food. We are taught early that "an apple a day keeps the doctor away." Children love apple juice and apple pie is synonymous with picnics, holidays, and home. Applesauce is a staple of the diets of children from a very young age. I remember being relieved when my young son, the carnivore, would eat applesauce because this was the only "fruit or vegetable" that he would ingest. So, imagine what would happen if this iconic fruit was threatened by a contaminant that could pose a risk to our health—or, more importantly, our children's health. If the potential health effect was identified as cancer, panic would likely ensue, apple markets would crumble, and angry parents would demand that the government strengthen regulations to protect their children from the risk.

This scenario played out in the late 1980s when the country became gripped in the throes of an apple catastrophe, complete with protests, legislative hearings, and celebrity activism. Schools across the country eliminated apples from their lunch menus and millions of apples were dumped because the American public was too scared to eat them. The fear arose from concerns over a chemical that was used by many growers to increase profitability of the apple crop and it was uncovered that this chemical was related to rocket fuel.

Rocket Fuel on Apples

The chemical culprit was Alar (chemical name daminozide), a growth hormone that was approved by the federal government in 1963 and subsequently became a major tool in the apple industry. The primary purpose of Alar was to extend the shelf life of apples, something that is extremely important to produce suppliers because of the seasonality of their product. The longer apples can last without getting rotten or looking bad, the farther they can be shipped and the more available they can be at all times of the year in every grocery store in America.

The federal government also approved Alar for use on cherries, peaches, pears, and Concord grapes, among other fruits, but it was the apple story that got the attention of environmental health activists and the media. Children eat and drink a lot of apple products, so the apple industry became a battleground in the fight to reduce risks from pesticides in our food supply. Apple juice is in most of the fruit juice blends that are marketed specifically to children. If you look closely at the labels of these products, you will find that apple juice concentrate is the first ingredient listed on juices that are marketed as white grape juice, peach mango juice, and numerous other flavors. In addition, most pediatricians recommend that apple juice be the first juice introduced in the diets of children because of its mild flavor and gentle laxative effect.[2]

When the federal government approved Alar in 1963 they did not know that they were approving a potential carcinogen. The problem wasn't the Alar itself, but the by-product of Alar, a chemical compound called unsymmetrical dimethylhydrazine (UDMH). Scientists discovered that UDMH could result from heat processing foods, thus creating an issue for apple sauce and apple juice producers. UDMH is one of a group of chemical compounds known as hydrazines; the chemical formula for UDMH is $C_2H_8N_2$. These compounds contain two nitrogen atoms joined by a single covalent bond that occurs when atoms share electrons as they bond together. Hydrazines are contained in a classification of chemicals known as amines and one of the distinguishing characteristics of amines is that they have a strong, foul odor.

UDMH has been used in rocket fuel; specifically in the rockets that carry heavy equipment to the International Space Station. During launch of these rockets, UDMH is released into the ambient environment, and preliminary studies in Kazakhstan suggest that there are significant environmental and human health effects as a result.[3] The idea of eating apples doused with rocket propellant is not only unappetizing; it is probably downright scary to most people.

How did the government approve the use of a chemical that could eventually turn into rocket fuel? The approval process is found in the law entitled the Federal Insecticide, Fungicide, and Rodenticide Act also known as FIFRA. FIFRA became law in 1947 and a major component of the law is a registration process for chemicals. In order for any new chemical to enter the market, the manufacturer must supply data to the EPA that include possible environmental and human health effects. Scientists at the EPA determine how to categorize the chemical based on these data. The data provided by the manufacturer indicated to the EPA that the chemical could be approved for use on foods. The standard for approval is that the chemical will not lead to "unreasonable adverse effects." In 1963 the EPA allowed Alar onto the market following the protocol laid out in FIFRA. At that time, the data available did not suggest that exposure to Alar would cause unreasonable adverse effects, so the EPA approved it for use on fruits.

Twenty-five years after its registration, Alar was condemned as a cancer-causing chemical thanks to the suspected carcinogen UDMH, the by-product associated with the breakdown of Alar. The science on the health effects of UDMH was incomplete during the late 1980s when the scare surfaced, and it is still incomplete today. However, there was enough evidence to convince many that UDMH could result from processing practices that heated foods treated with Alar. Once this became known to the public, there was an intense focus on the health of the nation's children and politicians had to get involved in order to be responsive to their constituents. In 1989, the manufacturer of Alar, Uniroyal, stopped producing Alar, and it only took about one year for Alar to become undetectable as a residue on apples.

Almost 10 years after Alar was pulled off the market, there was still no scientific consensus as to whether UDMH caused cancer. Scientists at the EPA said that it "probably" caused cancer. The DHHS said that it "may reasonably be anticipated" to cause cancer. The International Agency for Research on Cancer said that is "possibly" causes cancer. Finally, the American Conference of Governmental Industrial Hygienists believed that UDMH should be classified as an animal carcinogen only because it was not likely to cause cancer in humans unless they are exposed at high levels.[4] Regardless of the uncertainty, as soon as the chemical name and the word "cancer" are used in the same sentence, people pay attention and want to learn more about how to protect themselves and their families from exposure. In many cases, the public turns to the media for answers to their questions and the media played a major role on the Alar case.

The Controversy Comes to TV

The catalyzing event of the Alar scare occurred on CBS's *60 Minutes* in February 1989. The show opened with the following: "The most potent cancer-causing agent in our food supply is a substance sprayed on apples to keep them on the trees longer and make them look better. That's the conclusion of a number of scientific experts. And who is most at risk? Children, who may someday develop cancer from this one chemical called daminozide. Daminozide, which has been sprayed on apples for more than 20 years, breaks down into another chemical called UDMH."[5]

Who wouldn't be afraid when a respected news organization is calling the chemical that is on the fruit most beloved by children the "most potent cancer-causing agent" in the food supply? This was a story designed to alarm the public and to raise awareness about the use of chemicals in food production. The fallout from this broadcast was widespread, including economic damage to apple growers, a ban on the use of Alar in the food supply, and a lawsuit against CBS for the economic consequences of their story.

The Natural Resources Defense Council (NRDC) was the environmental health activist group that took the lead in getting the issue of Alar on apples into the news.[6] By many accounts, NRDC was thought to be in collusion with CBS by giving them an exclusive to the report, which was officially released by NRDC the day after the *60 Minutes* broadcast.[7] This approach to framing science in the media as opposed to using the standard peer review and publishing process is one that works very well for environmental health activists. It puts the organization that is releasing the information on the offensive and forces everyone else involved into a defensive position. So, Uniroyal, the Alar manufacturer, and the EPA, the government agency responsible for allowing the chemical in the food supply, had to explain why they would produce and allow this potent carcinogen to contaminate apples. Critics of the way in which the NRDC released the information and kept it in the press argued that the story had more to do with public relations than with scientific information about the environmental health risk.

Although the media was criticized for sensationalizing the story, one study that examined media coverage during 1989, the year that the story broke, found data that supported the opposite conclusion.[8] That is, in examining stories in major newspapers during the Alar scare, the researchers found that the print media was fair in their coverage of the story, giving reasonable opportunities to all sides. However, the print media did focus more on the controversy surrounding the nature of the debate rather than on the scientific uncertainties themselves. This study did not examine broadcast media coverage that included the *60 Minutes* piece and talk shows such as *Phil Donohue* covering the story.

The print media followed up the 1989 story with several accounts of the aftermath of the Alar scare. For example, the *New York Times* cover story on July 9, 1991, told the story of a family of apple farmers in Seattle, Washington, whose farm went into foreclosure because Americans were afraid to eat apples or products made with apples. According to the article, the USDA reported that apple farmers in the state of Washington lost more than $215 million in revenue immediately after Alar became synonymous with poisoned apples.

Celebrities Get Involved

The Alar case was one of the first to highlight the impact that celebrities can have on environmental health issues, specifically those related to the safety of the food supply. In 1989, Meryl Streep became a spokesperson for children's environmental health. She not only made public appeals to curb apple consumption, but she testified before U.S. Congress on the issue. To some, she was viewed as more credible than scientists at the EPA, and her opinion and celebrity heightened awareness, and fear, about the levels of pesticides on food. In an interview with *USA Today* in 2002, she admitted that she was a reluctant activist and that she was not prepared for the response she received from some groups as a result of her actions. She said, "the lawsuits that followed me, the irate growers, the people who broke into my home—I was really very intimidated by all that. I'm really more like Julia Roberts than Erin Brockovich."[9]

As is the case with many environmental issues, scientists continued to study the health effects of Alar after it was introduced into our food supply. The EPA was concerned enough about Alar that it was planning to ban its use on foods in May 1989 (subsequent to the *60 Minutes* broadcast), citing a link with cancers in laboratory animals.[10] The manufacturer, Uniroyal, headed off any mandatory ban of their product in their voluntarily removal of Alar from circulation in 1990. Public perception and fear were critical to the exclusion of this chemical from the food supply. The Alar scenario is an excellent example of the power of public perception. When people are scared, they demand action, and the government generally acts. It also demonstrates the lengths to which we will go to protect our children from uncertain environmental health threats, as well as the economic costs of fear.

Another Apple Poison Surfaces

The irony in the Alar controversy is that while it was receiving so much attention, an even more alarming contaminant could have been poisoning the same apples that were being used to make cider. *E. coli* O157:H7 was discovered in unpasteurized apple cider implicated in an outbreak in several states from 1996 to 1997. In the western United States, 66 people became ill and one person died from drinking unpasteurized cider or juice. A related outbreak in which more than 20 people were ill was identified in Connecticut not too long after confirmation of the outbreak in the west.[11]

Apples used in cider and some juices are generally collected from the ground because blemished apples will not sell as table fruit but are fine for pressing into cider. We are certain that *E. coli* lives in the intestines of animals, so the contamination of the cider was linked to the proximity of cattle to the orchards. When cattle use orchards for grazing, they may leave behind intestinal pathogens that get onto the fallen apples. If the apples are not washed well and the cider or juice isn't pasteurized, these pathogens can remain in the liquid and even grow at room temperature.

There were cases of severe illness related to consuming apple products contaminated with *E. coli*; however it will be difficult to ever identify specific cancer cases associated with Alar on apples. Another difference between the microbiological and chemical contamination of apples is that there was no major public outcry about the bacterial contamination of apples. Celebrities did not urge people to dump their apple cider or risk getting diarrhea, which is usually considered a much less serious and frightening disease than cancer. Congress never held a public hearing about *E. coli* in apple cider.

The Alar case underscores the fact that, at least at the time, we were much less concerned about giving our children acute diarrhea than we were about possibly increasing their risk of cancer at some undefined point in the future. The case also laid the foundation for similar food safety scares including one that surfaced at about the same time that the public discourse about Alar was fading into the background. This case is perhaps even scarier than Alar because of the scientific uncertainty that surrounds it and the fact that it involves another all-American food: the hamburger.

GROUND PROTEIN PATHOGENS

In 1995 in the United Kingdom, a strange thing happened. Three young men died of a rare neurological disease named after the two physicians who were responsible for first identifying its characteristics. The disease, known as Creutzfeldt-Jakob disease or CJD, is a frightening way to die. It involves a gradual loss of all motor control, including the inability of the body to operate all of its life-sustaining systems. One of the men who died was 19, the other was 28, and the third was 29. This was a very strange situation because of the nature of CJD; it is a disease that usually attacks older people and has rarely taken the life of anyone under the age of the age of 50.

In 1995, CJD was identified as the cause of death 47 times in the United Kingdom. Starting in 1995, the number of annual deaths increased steadily to a high of 108 in 2003. One possible explanation for the steady increase in CJD-related deaths was thought to be the relationship between an aging population and the long latency period of the disease. It can take years, even decades, for CJD to develop to the point that it becomes life-threatening. So as a greater proportion of the population passed middle age, the incidence of the disease was increasing according to expectations.

The deaths of three men under the age of 30 in 1995 perplexed scientists even further when they discovered that the brains of these three men looked different than brains in other CJD cases.[12] It was clear that while the cause of death was some type of encephalopathy, and similar to CJD, that there were distinct features about the brains of these three victims that were distinguishable from other documented CJD cases. This was the beginning what would become known as variant CJD or vCJD and the United Kingdom is considered ground zero for this illness. Several other countries reported cases of vCJD in the 1990s, but at least one study suggests that all roads lead to the United Kingdom as the likely source of all such cases.[13]

As scientists searched for the specific pathogen that caused vCJD, they began to focus on the food supply as a possible mode of transmission.

The most alarming difference between vCJD and CJD is the median age at which the disease appears in people. For vCJD, the median age of onset is 26 and of death, 28. Previously recorded cases of normal CJD identify the median age of onset as 66, and death at 67. About 10 years before the first deaths related to vCJD were discovered in the young people in the United Kingdom, a similar illness had reached near-epidemic proportions in the cattle industry. The illness in cattle was referred to as mad cow disease because of the way that animals behaved when stricken by the illness; they lost control of all their motor functions including their ability to stand.

In 1998, mad cow disease was referred to as "one of the greatest human-made disasters in history."[14] It was also suggested that it was similar to the Exxon Valdez oil spill, Chernobyl, and the Bhopal disaster in that it was preventable, caused by humans, and led to severe economic consequences. In addition, this illness was scary because of the uncertainty related to its cause, and the possibility that it was being transmitted to humans, leading to the new variation in CJD.

What's In a Name?

CJD is not a new disease; it was identified in the 1920s by two German neurologists, Hans Gerhard Creutzfeldt and Alfons Maria Jakob. Creutzfeldt and Jakob were very different people in terms of their personalities, lifestyles, and scientific interpretation of the human cases that they studied. Rather than CJD being identified based on collaborative research, it appears that it was a political move that has linked them forever in the name of the illness that they both found fascinating.

Creutzfeldt was born in 1885 in Harburg, Germany. His family had a medical background so he was raised with an awareness of science and medicine. He had strong political opinions and was an outspoken critic of Nazism. He served in the German navy during World War I and during World War II he lost his home and clinic to bombing. Even though he criticized Hitler, and his wife went to jail for her similar opinions, he was insulated from harassment because of his connection to the German navy. He was a doctor in the German navy during World War II, and some of the men he served with during World War I were high-ranking officials. His experience and connections are reportedly the reason why he was not imprisoned or harmed by the Third Reich despite his views about Hitler and the Nazis.[15]

In 1913, Creutzfeldt was working in a clinic attending to patients with severe neurological problems. At this time, there was a woman in the clinic who exhibited behavioral conditions different from any other mental conditions he had ever observed. The standard scientific method would have led Creutzfeldt to publish his observations to share with the wider scientific community. However, he was delayed in publishing an account of this case due to his World War I military service. It wasn't until 1920 that he was able to publish the case and his paper drew the interest of another German neuropathologist, Alfons Jakob.

Jakob was born in Bavaria in 1884 and spent his childhood helping his father tend to the family shop. Unlike Creutzfeldt, Jakob was reportedly a private person, but with a stellar reputation in his field.[16] Even though their public personae were different, Creutzfeldt and Jakob had several things in common. They both trained in the same clinic in Munich, and both of them worked with Alois Alzheimer, a name that needs no explanation today. Jakob died in 1931 at the age of 47, 34 years before the death of Creutzfeldt.

In 1920 Jakob read Creutzfeldt's papers about the unusual neurological disease that took the life of a 22-year-old woman at Alzheimer's clinic. The written history of this patient was completed in great detail and included behavioral observations and a description of her brain as it appeared during an autopsy. One of Creutzfeldt's papers about this case also presents a daily journal of the patient and "a remarkable dialogue between a dying demented woman and a compassionate physician."[17] Jakob identified several cases similar to what Creutzfeldt described; however, Creutzfeldt was critical of how Jakob described the illness.

It appears as if Creutzfeldt and Jakob never formally collaborated on researching this condition. The name Creutzfeldt-Jakob disease was attributed to Walther Spielmeyer, another well-known neuropathologist of the time, who coined the term in a seemingly political move to promote his school, which was competing with Jakob's. Spielmeyer held mutual views with Creutzfeldt and shared a close relationship with him as well. He probably understood the significance of Creutzfeldt's and Jakob's work and spoke of the disease using Creutzfeldt's name first to ensure the posterity of his colleague.

Creutzfeld and Jakob never used the term to describe their work, nor did they allow their students to do so.[18] There was also some controversy over whether what they had discovered was a disease that could be attributed to a cause or a syndrome that could be the result of multiple causes. They both died, decades apart, believing that they were researching a syndrome rather than a specific disease.

The Animal Version

"Mad cow" is the term applied to the disease similar to CJD in cattle. Also known as bovine spongiform encephalopathy (BSE), this condition has been identified as a disease that is transmissible from animal to animal. Even though BSE was only identified in the mid-1980s, a similar disorder called "scrapie" has been noted in sheep for at least 250 years.[19] BSE and scrapie belong to a group called transmissible spongiform encephalopathies (TSEs). Other TSEs include "chronic wasting disease" in wild animals and a specific type of disease that affects only mink.

Scrapie is found across the globe, including the United States. As of 2004, only Australia and New Zealand were recognized as being free of the disease. In the case of scrapie, the disease-causing organism is thought to be transmitted from ewes to their lambs through the placenta. The first case of scrapie in the United States was identified in Michigan in 1947. To get a sense of the scale of the problem of scrapie in the United States, the USDA's Animal and Plant Health Inspection Service (APHIS) published a report in 2004 estimating that only about 0.20 percent of the sheep in the United States may be infected.[20]

Genetics has a role to play in the susceptibility of sheep to scrapie, and some species of sheep are not likely to get the disease, whereas others are highly susceptible. Even though the incidence of scrapie in the United States is estimated to be very low, the U.S. government enacted rules restricting interstate commerce involving sheep.[21] These rules require that all sheep and goats that will be crossing state lines be properly identified with an ear tag or a stamp. In addition, there must be a Certificate of Veterinary Inspection accompanying each animal. The certificate is required to verify that the animals are free of scrapie. The purpose of the regulations is to stop the spread of the disease by ensuring that all animals that are moving around the country are healthy.

Identifying the Cause

Research related to CJD has progressed at a rapid rate since the early 1920s; however, there is still some disagreement about the cause of the illness. Microbiologists have searched for bacteria and viruses as the causes and have continued to come up empty-handed. The theory that emerged in the 1980s was that the illness was caused by a protein that defied all techniques used to control other microbiological pathogens. This protein was labeled a "prion."

Prion is short for "proteinaceous infectious particle." Unlike bacteria and viruses, prions cannot be eliminated from foods by cooking, even at high temperatures. Dr. Stanley Prusiner, a neurologist at the University of California San Francisco, is credited with the discovery of the prion and in

1997 he won the Nobel Prize in Physiology or Medicine for his discovery. Prusiner identified the prion as the potential cause of TSEs in 1984 and since then, millions of dollars of research has resulted in hundreds of papers about prions and their relationship to TSE.

Despite all of this research, there are still numerous unanswered questions about prions. For example, another potential problem with prions is a lack of understanding of how they act in the environment. There is evidence that they can survive in soil for extended periods of time, which could be a contributing factor to chronic wasting disease in wild animals. However, there is not enough research to provide an adequate understanding of how prions might act in landfills or even in wastewater.[22] Perhaps we are being exposed to prions in many ways in the environment, not just by eating a hamburger.

Because routine sterilization techniques do not work on prions, there is concern with spreading them in institutional environments. This is especially the case in facilities that offer medical procedures on the brain including biopsies and surgery. In December 2007, a hospital near Milwaukee, Wisconsin, was involved in a CJD scare. A patient had a brain biopsy and after the biopsy the hospital suspected that this patient might be suffering from CJD. If CJD was suspected prior to the biopsy, special precautions would have been taken to minimize the potential for spreading the suspected prions to other patients. No precautions were taken for this particular patient, so the hospital reacted by canceling all surgeries for several hours so that surgical equipment could be re-sterilized with methods that kill prions. The hospital took this measure and held press conferences to assure the public that the risk was "infinitesimally small."[23]

The Wisconsin hospital case underscores the belief by many in the scientific community that prions are the cause of CJD. However, there are scientists who are still skeptical about the link between prions and CJD. In 2007, researchers at Yale University presented evidence that prions might not be the real culprits in TSEs.[24] They examined a strain of TSE found in sheep and a CJD strain that is found in humans. The researchers explained that even though there have been 25 years of research focusing on prions as the cause of the diseases, there has been no evidence that prions are infectious. In the course of their research, they found evidence of viral particles in addition to the prions. As a result, they argue that the presence of a virus is a "clear, consistent, substantive, and logical alternative to the accepted prion hypothesis."[25]

The Hamburger Link

Because the cattle version of TSE was so similar to vCJD in terms of both the clinical presentation and the characteristics of the brain upon autopsy, researchers began to speculate about the link between animals and humans to explain vCJD. Because it was generally accepted that mad cow disease and scrapie could be transmissible from animal to animal, a hypothesis emerged that the illness could be transmitted from animals to humans. This hypothesis has been the driving force behind a substantial body of research for more than a quarter of a century. Even though the Nobel Prize–winning Prusiner was relatively certain that prions were causing CJD in humans, in his own words, he was "initially dubious of the presumed link between BSE and vCJD."[26] He said he changed his mind after so many studies, most using laboratory mice, indicated that there was a relationship between the two.

Hamburger has been implicated as one culprit in the spread of the disease in humans, in contrast to steaks or roasts or other muscle meat, which are of little worry. This is because prions have been found only in the brains and spinal cords of animals and these components of the animals may find their way into ground beef. To further implicate consumption of animal brains as the cause of vCJD, researchers have examined cases of a disease known as kuru that was widespread in Papua New Guinea in the 1950s. According to historical accounts from specific communities in this part of the world, cannibalism was part of the funeral ritual when a member of the community died, a ritual dating back to at least the 1920s. Men were given the first choice of the cadaver, leaving parts such as the brains to women, and in some instances, children. Incidence of kuru was more common in women than men, and since the cannibalistic ritual stopped in the 1950s, the incidence of any documented cases of kuru has declined substantially.

In 1996, a team of researchers went to Papua New Guinea in search of kuru cases and only found 11 from 1996 to 2004. Since cannibalism stopped in the 1950s, and the infected cases were all born before it stopped, the researchers concluded that kuru could have a longer incubation period than was previously thought. It is possible, they said, that this illness, which is clinically similar to vCJD, could incubate in the human body for 40 or more years.[27] This type of research is alarming in that it suggests that, if there is a connection between consuming contaminated meat and vCJD, there may be many more cases of vCJD yet to come. In addition, as our population ages and we see more cases of neurological diseases such as Alzheimer's and dementia, it is likely that research will continue to examine the possible link between food and these illnesses. Other researchers have already suggested that meat consumption might be a major contributing factor in Alzheimer's disease as well as vCJD.[28]

Perhaps the situation with mad cow disease was summed up best by a former U.S. government official. When presenting a brief history of BSE in cattle, Lester Crawford, a veterinarian who was briefly the commissioner of the FDA, said, "The great lesson of the BSE event is that the world of bacteria, viruses, and prions are in fiendish conspiracy to decimate or even extinguish higher life forms. Moreover, there is contained in the ever-evolving pool of genetic tricks available to that unseen world, the capacity to cause heretofore uncontemplated havoc to each other, to humans and to any other non-human life forms."[29]

The Bottom Line

Despite all of the research and the major concerns raised by the public health community and environmental health activists, the mad cow story is similar to the Alar story in that, to date, the greatest damages caused by mad cow disease do not appear to have been inflicted on public health. Rather, the greatest damages are economic, social, and political in nature. Results have included a reduction in beef consumption, the slaughter of millions of animals, new restrictive policies on blood and organ donations, and a potential international trade crisis.

Public perception of risk is the catalyzing agent for all of the responses to both Alar and mad cow disease. In both of these cases, people became afraid because of the nature of the risks. There has been considerable research examining factors that contribute to public perception of risk. When the risk is viewed as involuntary, exotic, human-made, catastrophic, and dreaded, people's fears are heightened to levels that will translate into specific behaviors. The offending product or agent may be stigmatized to the point that people avoid exposure. In addition, when public fears are high, citizens demand answers from their governments as to why they were not protected from exposure.

Concerns over mad cow disease affected the bottom line of beef producers and restaurants. One study of the effect of the perception of risk from mad cow disease in France documented that the more afraid and worried people were about the disease, the less beef they consumed.[30] At the height of the crisis in the United Kingdom, individual restaurants saw an immediate decline in profit from menu items containing beef. This was due to a typical consumer behavior in the face of fear, one of product avoidance.[31] As restaurants in Europe were suffering from a decline in beef-related business, the agriculture community was bearing an even greater cost. In Europe more than 5 million cattle were destroyed to address the spread of BSE. Entire herds were sacrificed and farmers lost everything.

On April 4, 2001, the U.S. Senate Committee on Commerce, Science, and Transportation held a hearing to discuss mad cow disease. The hearing was entitled, "Mad Cow Disease: Are Our Precautions Adequate?"[32] Most of the senators who made statements at this hearing recognized that there was never a single case of variant CJD recorded in the United States. In addition, at that time, there also had not been a case of BSE reported. Many of the senators also mentioned a *Newsweek* article that focused on mad cow disease.

One of the major challenges of protecting the U.S. food supply from BSE was summed up at the hearing by Stephen Sundlof, who was the director of the Center of Veterinary Medicine at the FDA during this time. When describing the role of the federal government, Sundlof noted that there were four components to the approach of the federal government: (1) surveillance, (2) protection, (3) research, and (4) oversight. This is easier said than done given the fact that these activities are decentralized as described by Sundlof during the hearing, "Surveillance for human disease is primarily the responsibility of CDC. Protection and surveillance of animals, feeds and foods are responsibilities of the FDA, which it shares with USDA. Research is primarily the responsibility of NIH, although FDA conducts important research. Oversight is primarily the responsibility of the DHHS Office of the Secretary."[33]

A lack of coordination was evident as the U.S. mad cow disease situation played out a little differently than it did in Europe. The first cow to be positively identified as having BSE was found on a farm in the state of Washington in December 2003. The economic reaction to this discovery was swift, as other countries immediately banned beef imported from the United States. The United States also banned importation of animals from Canada after it was determined that this was where the sick cow was from. There were so many bans of beef trade at this time that it was difficult to keep track of all of them.

According to the Government Accountability Office (GAO), while the first BSE case had economic consequences in terms of the U.S. ability to export beef, it did not hurt domestic American beef consumption.[34] Japan, which was the largest consumer of American beef, banned all imports of beef from the United States. Meanwhile in the United States, beef consumption has steadily increased, a trend thought to be encouraged by the popularity of high-protein diets. One could conclude that Americans are more interested in losing weight than in avoiding a fatal, brain-wasting disease.

The U.S. government has three basic strategies that have been employed to address BSE: (1) a ban on live animal imports from countries with any BSE; (2) surveillance of live cattle; and (3) a ban on feed that contains animal parts. According to the GAO, the most important component of the FDA's plan is the feed ban. In 2005, the GAO issued a report that was highly critical of the way in which the FDA was managing the feed ban.[35] In order for the ban to be successful, facilities that produce cattle feed, sources of the raw materials for the feed, transportation companies that haul the feed, and the farms that provide the feed to their animals must be held accountable.

In the United States, to keep industry accountable, we generally require inspections and paperwork. According to the FDA, almost 15,000 facilities are subject to the feed ban and should comply with inspections and record-keeping procedures. In 2004, the FDA was able to inspect only about 6,000 facilities.

The GAO explained that there were serious deficiencies in the inspections that the FDA did conduct. Essentially, the FDA was being too lenient on the firms by not following up when problems were identified, by not diligently enforcing compliance with the law, and by misrepresenting compliance levels to the public and elected officials. One of the major problems is that the FDA does not know where all of the facilities that might be subject to the ban are located. FDA personnel told the GAO that they "looked through phone books" as a way to identify potential facilities.[36]

The greatest concern raised in the GAO report was that when the FDA identified that cattle had been fed banned feed, they did not contact the USDA. The USDA could have monitored the cattle that were fed the bogus feed for signs of BSE. So, since the 2001 hearing in which coordination issues were highlighted by and to members of Congress, there have been ongoing problems with the system for keeping the U.S. food supply free of BSE. Monitoring the feed ban is just one example of the lack of coordination among agencies involved in controlling mad cow disease.

Aside from the issues with tracking feed, another problem with compliance is emerging in research being conducted in France. One study has identified almost 1,000 cows with BSE that have been born after France banned contaminated feed in 1990.[37] It appears that farmers, and the government, have a difficult time ensuring that feed intended for cattle has not been cross-contaminated during manufacture in facilities that process feed for other types of animals.

Global Impact

As noted above, countries with any documented cases of BSE in their cattle became global pariahs when it came to trade in beef products. Other countries would not import anything containing beef and, in most cases, animals were slaughtered and destroyed if there was any suspicion of BSE in the herd. The international trade consequences and economic fallout that resulted from mad cow disease are the major reason why the mad cow situation can be called a "crisis."

Immediately after the first case of BSE was found in cattle in the United States, the Japanese government banned American beef from their country. This was a major economic hit to American beef producers, who reportedly exported about $1.4 billion worth of beef to Japan in 2003 alone. Overall, between 2003 and 2004, U.S. exports of beef and beef products declined 79 percent from about $3.8 billion in 2003 to just over $800 million in 2004. The situation improved between 2004 and 2005 due to increased trade with Canada, the Middle East, and Vietnam. The Japanese ban remained in effect until 2006 when it was lifted following political pressure from the United States.

In late 2005, Japan and the United States reached an agreement that would lift the ban and importations of U.S. beef into Japan resumed. Trade continued for about six weeks until a mistake made by a meatpacking company in Brooklyn accidentally shipped beef that contained a spinal column to Japan. Japan immediately instituted another ban, meaning that one meatpacking company in Brooklyn was able to shut down the entire U.S. beef export industry once again.

The situation improved somewhat in 2006 when Japan again relaxed the ban. According to the U.S. Meat Export Federation, beef exports from the United States to Japan increased 440 percent between 2006 and 2007. Although this was a major increase, the value of the exports was estimated at about $194 million, well below the billions being exported prior to 2003. It may take many more years for the beef industry in the United States to recover from the scare of mad cow disease, and it will only take one more confirmed case in the United States to further erode any trust that may now be rebuilding between the United States and Japan.

In November 2007, the USDA reached an agreement with the Canadian government to resume importation of products that were banned in 2003. According to the memo issued by the USDA on November 14, 2007, the agreement allowed the United States to import most formerly prohibited products both with and without an import permit. Products allowed to be imported without a permit must be certified safe by the Canadian Food Inspection Agency and include beef, sheep, and goat and products such as casings for sausages, as long as the involved animals were slaughtered before they were 12 months old. Other products that could be imported without a permit were those containing bone and gelatin. All other beef products require a permit, including pet foods that contain animal products, and animal feeds that contain animal products. Regardless of whether a permit is required, the Canadian imports must enter the United States at specific sites so that federal officials can inspect them.

How was the United States able to resume exports of beef less than two years after the first case of BSE was documented in the country? This is an especially interesting question because it took almost 10 years for the ban on beef from the United Kingdom to be lifted by the European Union (EU). The United Kingdom was banned from exporting beef in 1996, and in 2006, the EU lifted this ban and exports to other EU countries resumed, even though some countries, notably France and Germany, remained reluctant to accept beef from the United Kingdom. As of late 2007, the United States still does not import beef from the United Kingdom.

An illuminating account of the U.S. role in global beef markets under siege by BSE comes from an Australian perspective.[38] Whereas the U.S. GAO notes the three-pronged U.S. approach of surveillance, bans on imported beef, and bans on specific feeds, Australian policy analysts suggest a different three-pronged approach adopted in the United States in the realm of global trade. This approach includes: (1) defending and promoting an image of the United States as being a country with no significant risk of BSE; (2) working vigorously to change international standards to suit its own interests; and (3) making the voluntary international standards mandatory so that other countries are required to comply with them.[39]

In a nutshell, when it comes to involvement in global beef trade, the United States has been perceived as a bully. This bully status played out in 2004 as the United States and Australia negotiated a Free Trade Agreement (FTA). In a strange move, a "side letter" was appended to the FTA that, while ambiguously written, seems to compel Australia to further U.S. interests to resume beef exports. This was very strange because Australia was considered a "BSE-free" country and the letter suggested that they would allow imports of U.S. beef to resume.

Hamburgers and Oprah

In addition to the international trade ramifications, the mad cow crisis was, and continues to be, a communication crisis.[40] The same author who referred to mad cow disease as "one of the greatest human-made disasters in history," wrote an editorial in 2006 noting that the human health impacts of the disease have not materialized as first feared. This editorial comes 10 years after one of the most influential people in the world swore off hamburgers.

The *Oprah* show that aired in April 1996 was designed to be a show about dangerous food in general, but it turned into a show that focused on mad cow disease. According to the legal proceedings from the case that was brought by the Cattlemen's Association,[41] the edited show that ultimately aired did not contain several minutes of commentary by the food experts noting that the risk of acquiring the human variant of mad cow disease in the United States was almost zero. Also deleted was discussion about the safety of the food supply in the United States and comments made by the activist agreeing that the beef in America is generally safe to eat.

The situations with Alar and with mad cow disease are similar in that important public figures weighed in on the safety of the food supply. The result was a heightened level of public awareness that translated into economic consequences for the food suppliers. When members of the public are afraid, in addition to doing whatever they can to avoid the thing they are afraid of, they often will demand that the government take steps to minimize their risk. So, elected officials hold well-orchestrated hearings and create legislation that is often meaningless, but at least officials give the appearance that something is being done. These hearings are in the news for a short period of time, and as soon as the next major public health scare surfaces, the focus shifts and people forget about why they were holding hearings in the first place.

The reactionary approach on the part of our government to very specific threats has created a fragmented food safety system that may not be capable of handling unexpected problems. We have seen many unexpected problems illustrated by the outbreaks that have been discussed in this book. When government agencies that are supposed to be responsible for ensuring safe food have to accommodate the public scare of the moment, it is not possible to perform competent planning or preparation. Managing by the public fear du jour, or crisis management, does not allow us to address the most important invaders in our food supply, the microbiological contaminants.

While we have had our attention diverted by the potential risks of terrorism, nuclear war, and pandemic influenza, bacteria and viruses have been quietly infecting our food supply. They have also been evolving to withstand our traditional approaches to killing them. Hopefully with a greater understanding of how these pathogens survive in food and how they can make you sick, you will be able to focus as a consumer, and as your own last line of defense on protecting your health. Let's dream of a world in which you never suffer from diarrhea again.

NOTES

1. Howard Lyman on the *Oprah Winfrey Show*, April 15, 1996, transcript, http://www.vegsource.com/lyman/oprah_transcript.htm.

2. Apple Products Research and Education Council, "Frequently Asked Questions about Fruit Juice," http://www.appleproducts.org/qanda.html.

3. Lars Carlsen, Olga A. Kenesova, and Svetlana E. Batyrbekova, "A Preliminary Assessment of the Potential Environmental and Human Health Impact of Unsymmetrical Dimethylhydrazine as a Result of Space Activities," *Chemosphere* 67 (2007): 1108–16.

4. Agency for Toxic Substances and Disease Registry, "Public Health Profile for Hydrazines" (September 1997), http://www.atsdr.cdc.gov/toxprofiles/phs100.html.

5. *AUVIL v. CBS "60 MINUTES,"* 67 F.3d 816 (1995); *cert. denied* 116 S. Ct. 1567 (1996).

6. Natural Resources Defense Council, "Intolerable Risk: Pesticides in Our Children's Food" (February 27, 1989), http://tobaccodocuments.org/pm/2025546150-6160.html (accessed January 17, 2008).

7. Jay Lehr and Sam Aldrich, "Alar: The Great Apple Scare," *Environment News*, March 1, 2007; *The Wall Street Journal,* "How a PR Firm Executed the Alar Scare," October 3, 1989, Section 1, p. 22; Center for Media and Democracy, "One Bad Apple? Facts and Myths Behind the 'Alar Scare,'" *PR Watch Newsletter,* second quarter 1997, http://www.prwatch.org/prwissues/1997Q2/alar.html.

8. Sharon Friedman et al., "Alar and Apples: Newspapers, Risk and Media Responsibility," *Public Understanding of Science* 5 (1996): 1–20.

9. Adele Slaughter, "Meryl Streep Takes a Lead in Environmental Health," *USA Today*, October 18, 2002, http://www.usatoday.com/news/health/spotlighthealth/2002-10-18-streep-healthy-kids_x.htm.

10. U.S. EPA, "Daminozide (Alar) Pesticide Canceled for Food Uses," press release, November 7, 1989, http://www.epa.gov/history/topics/food/02.htm.

11. CDC, "Outbreaks of Escherichia coli O157:H7 Infection and Cryptosporidiosis Associated with Drinking Unpasteurized Apple Cider—Connecticut and New York, October 1996," *Morbidity and Mortality Weekly Report* 46, no. 01 (1997): 4–8, http://www.cdc.gov/mmwr/preview/mmwrhtml/00045558.htm.

12. R. G. Will and J. W. Ironside, "A New Variant of Creutzfeldt-Jakob in the UK," *The Lancet* 347 (1996): 921–25.

13. Pascual Sanchez-Juan et al., "Source of Variant Creutzfeldt-Jakob Disease outside the United Kingdom," *Emerging Infectious Diseases* 13, no. 8 (2007): 1166–68.

14. Scott C. Ratzan, *The Mad Cow Crisis* (New York: New York University Press, 1998), ix.

15. Serge Duckett and Jan Stern, "Origins of the Creutzfeldt and Jakob Concept," *Journal of the History of the Neurosciences* 8, no. 1 (1999): 21–34.

16. Ibid.

17. Ibid., 24.

18. Ibid.

19. Animal and Plant Health Inspection Service, "Scrapie," http://www.aphis.usda.gov/lpa/pubs/fsheet_faq_notice/fs_ahscrapie.html.

20. USDA, *NAHMS Scrapie: Ovine Slaughter Surveillance (SOSS) Study 2001–2003,* http://www.aphis.usda.gov/animal_health/animal_diseases/scrapie/downloads/sossphase2.pdf.

21. "Scrapie in Sheep and Goats; Interstate Movement Restrictions and Indemnity Program; Final Rule," *Federal Register* 66, no. 162 (August 21, 2001).

22. Joel A. Pedersen, Katherine D. McMahon, and Craig H. Benson, "Prions: Novel Pathogens of Environmental Concern?" *Journal of Environmental Engineering* (2006): 967–69.

23. Television interview with Dr. David Letzer, infectious disease specialist at Waukesha Memorial Hospital.

24. Laura Manuelidis et al. "Cells Infected with Scrapie and Creutzfeldt-Jakob Disease Agents Produce Intracellular 25-nm Virus-Like Particles," *Proceedings of the National Academy of Sciences* 104, no. 6 (2007): 1965–70.

25. Ibid., 1970.

26. Stanley B. Prusiner, "Detecting Mad Cow Disease," *Scientific American* 291, no. 1 (2004): 88.

27. John Collinge et al., "Kuru in the 21st Century—An Acquired Human Prion Disease with Very Long Incubation Periods," *The Lancet* 367 (2006): 2068–74.

28. Lawrence Broxmeyer, "Thinking the Unthinkable: Alzheimer's, Creutzfeld-Jakob and Mad Cow Disease: The Age-Related Reemergence of Virulent, Foodborne, Bovine Tuberculosis or Losing Your Mind for the Sake of a Shake or Burger," *Medical Hypothesis* 64 (2005): 699–705.

29. Lester M. Crawford, "BSE: A Veterinary History," in *The Mad Cow Crisis,* ed. Scott E. Ratzan, 14.

30. Michel Setbon et al., "Risk Perception of the 'Mad Cow Disease' in France: Determinant and Consequences," *Risk Analysis* 25, no. 4 (2005): 813–26.

31. Dennis Reynolds and William M. Balinbin, "Mad Cow Disease: An Empirical Investigation of Restaurant Strategies and Consumer Response," *Journal of Hospitality & Tourism Research* 27, no. 3 (2003): 358–68.

32. Senate Committee on Science, Commerce, and Transportation, *Mad Cow Disease: Are Our Precautions Adequate?* 107th Cong., 1st sess. (2001), http://bulk.resource.org/gpo.gov/hearings/107s/88461.pdf.

33. Ibid.

34. Government Accountability Office, *Mad Cow Disease: FDA's Management of the Feed Ban Has Improved, but Oversight Weaknesses Continue to Limit Program Effectiveness* (Washington, DC: GAO, 2005).

35. Ibid.

36. Ibid., 18.

37. Mathilde Paul et al., "Bovine Spongiform Encephalopathy and Spatial Analysis of the Feed Industry," *Emerging Infectious Diseases* 13, no. 6 (2007), http://www.cdc.gov/eid/content/13/6/contents_v13n06.htm.

38. Linda Weiss, Elizabeth Thurbon, and John Mathews, "Free Trade in Mad Cows: How to Kill a Beef Industry," *Australian Journal of International Affairs* 60, no. 1 (2006): 376–99.

39. Ibid.

40. See for example, Scott C. Ratzan, ed., *The Mad Cow Crisis*; William Leiss and Douglas Powell, *Mad Cows and Mother's Milk: The Perils of Poor Risk Communication* (Quebec: McGill-Queen's University Press, 2004).

41. *Texas Beef Group v. Oprah Winfrey*, 201 F.3d 680, ★; 2000 U.S. App. LEXIS 1723, 45 Fed. R. Serv. 3d (Callaghan) 1370.

Bibliography and Further Reading

Agasan, Alice, John Kornblum, George Williams, Chi-Chi Pratt, Phylis Fleckenstein, Marie Wong, and Alex Ramon. "Profile of *Salmonella enterica* subsp. *enterica* (subspecies I) serotype 4, 5, 12:i:- Strains Causing Foodborne Infection in New York City." *Journal of Clinical Microbiology* 40 (2002): 1924–29.

Agency for Toxic Substances and Disease Registry. "Public Health Profile for Hydrazines." September 1997. http://www.atsdr.cdc.gov/toxprofiles/phs100.html.

Ali, S. Harris. "A Socio-ecological Autopsy of the *E. coli O157:H7* Outbreak in Walkerton, Ontario, Canada." *Social Sciences & Medicine* 58 (2004): 2601–12.

Amon, J. J., R. Devasia, G. Xia, O. V. Nainan, S. Hall, B. Lawson, J. S. Wolthuis, P. D. Macdonald, C. W. Shepard, I. T. Williams, et al. "Molecular Epidemiology of Foodborne Hepatitis A Outbreaks in the United States, 2003." *The Journal of Infectious Diseases* 192 (2005): 1323–30.

Animal and Plant Health Inspection Service. "Scrapie." http://www.aphis.usda.gov/lpa/pubs/fsheet_faq_notice/fs_ahscrapie.html.

Apple Products Research and Education Council. "Frequently Asked Questions about Fruit Juice." http://www.appleproducts.org/qanda.html.

Armstrong, Gregory L., Jill Hollingsworth, and J. Glenn Morris, Jr. "Emerging Foodborne Pathogens: *E. coli* O157:H7 as a Model of the Entry of a New Pathogen into the Food Supply of the Developed World." *Epidemiologic Reviews* 18, no. 1 (1996): 29–51.

Avery, Donald H. *The Science of War: Canadian Scientists and Allied Military Technology During the Second World War* (Toronto: University of Toronto Press, 1998).

Basnyat, Buddha, A. P. Maskey, M. D. Zimmerman, and D. R. Murdoch. "Enteric (Typhoid) Fever in Travelers." *Clinical Infectious Diseases* 41 (2005): 1467–72.

Basu, Paroma. "Iraq's Public Health Infrastructure a Casualty of War." *Nature Medicine* 10, no. 2 (2004): 110.

Beck, Raymond W. *The Chronology of Microbiology in Historical Context.* (Washington, DC: ASM Press, 2000).

Benjamin, Elisabeth R., C. Clements, M. McCally, P. L. Pellett, M. J. Van Rooyen, and R. J. Wald-
man. "The Humanitarian Cost of a War in Iraq." *The Lancet* 361, no. 9360 (2003): 874.

Bentivoglio, Marina, and Paolo Pacini. "Filippo Pacini: A Determine Observer." *Brain Research
Bulletin* 38, no. 2 (1995): 161–65.

Beverage Marketing Corporation. *The 2004 Beverage Marketing Directory, Twenty-Sixth Edition*
(New York: Beverage Marketing Corporation, 2004).

Bhunia, Arun K. *Foodborne Microbial Pathogens: Mechanisms and Pathogenesis* (New York: Springer,
2008).

Bolton, D. J., A. Meally, D. McDowell, and I. S. Blair. "A Survey for Serotyping, Antibiotic
Resistance Profiling and PFGE Characterization of and the Potential Multiplication of
Restaurant *Salmonella* Isolates." *Journal of Applied Microbiology* 103 (2007): 1681–90.

Brannigan, Martha. "Widow Sues Carnival Alleging Wrongful Death." *The Miami Herald,*
October 26, 2006, Business and Financial News.

Broxmeyer, Lawrence. "Thinking the Unthinkable: Alzheimer's, Creutzfeld-Jakob and Mad Cow
Disease: The Age-Related Reemergence of Virulent, Foodborne, Bovine Tuberculosis
or Losing Your Mind for the Sake of a Shake or Burger." *Medical Hypothesis* 64 (2005):
699–705.

Buchanan, R. E., Ralph St. John-Brooks, and Robert S. Breed, eds. "International Bacteriological
Code of Nomenclature." *Journal of Bacteriology* 55, no. 3 (1948): 287–306.

Buck, Eugene H. "Hurricane Katrina Fishing and Aquaculture Industries—Damage and Recovery." *CRS Report for Congress.* September 7, 2005. http://www.fas.org/sgp/crs/misc/
RS22241.pdf.

Bureau of Labor Statistics. "Highest Incidence Rates of Total Nonfatal Occupational Injury and
Illness Cases, Private Industry, 2005." http://www.bls.gov/iif/oshwc/osh/os/ostb1607.
pdf.

Burnett, S. L., E. R. Gehm, W. R. Weissinger, and L. R. Beuchat. "Survival of *Salmonella* in Peanut Butter and Peanut Butter Spread." *Journal of Applied Microbiology* 89 (2000): 472–77.

Bush, George W. *Executive Order Creating Interagency Working Group on Import Safety.* 2007. http://
www.whitehouse.gov/news/releases/2007/07/20070718-4.html.

Butzler, J. P. "*Campylobacter,* from Obscurity to Celebrity." *Clinical Microbiology & Infection* 10
(2004): 868–76.

Campbell, K. J., and K. D. Hesketh. "Strategies Which Aim to Positively Impact on Weight,
Physical Activity, Diet and Sedentary Behaviours in Children from Zero to Five Years: A
Systematic Review of the Literature." *Obesity Reviews* 8 (2007): 327–38.

Capita, R., C. Alonso-Calleja, and M. Prieto. "Prevalence of *Salmonella enterica* Serovars and Genovars from Chicken Carcasses in Slaughterhouses in Spain." *Journal of Applied Microbiology*
103 (2007): 1366–75.

Carlsen, Lars, Olga A. Kenesova, and Svetlana E. Batyrbekova. "A Preliminary Assessment of the
Potential Environmental and Human Health Impact of Unsymmetrical Dimethylhydrazine as a Result of Space Activities." *Chemosphere* 67 (2007): 1108–16.

Carter, J. D., and L. R. Espinoza. "Interplay of Environmental Triggers and Host Response in
Reactive Arthritis: Can We Intervene?" *Future Rheumatology* 1 (2006): 717–27.

Centers for Disease Control and Prevention. "Achievements in Public Health, 1900–1999: Safer
and Healthier Foods." *Morbidity and Mortality Weekly Reports* 48, no. 40 (1999), http://
www.cdc.gov/mmwr/preview/mmwrhtml/mm4840a1.htm.

———. "Botulism Associated with Commercially Canned Chili Sauce—Texas and Indiana,
July 2007." *Morbidity and Mortality Weekly Reports* 56, no. 30 (2007): 467–69, http://www.
cdc.gov/mmwr/preview/mmwrhtml/mm5630a4.htm.

———. "Compendium of Measures to Prevent Disease Associated with Animals in Public
Settings, 2007." *Morbidity and Mortality Weekly Report* 56, no. RR05 (2007): 1–13, http://
www.cdc.gov/mmwr/preview/mmwrhtml/rr5605a1.htm.

————. "Extensively Drug-Resistant Tuberculosis." http://www.cdc.gov/tb/XDRTB/default. htm (accessed January 8, 2008).

————. "Fruit and Vegetable Consumption Among Adults—United States, 2005." *Morbidity and Mortality Weekly Report* 56, no. 10 (2007), http://www.cdc.gov/mmwr/preview/ mmwrhtml/mm5610a2.htm.

————. "Multisite Outbreak of Norovirus Associated with a Franchise Restaurant—Kent County, Michigan, May 2005." *Morbidity and Mortality Weekly Reports* 55 (2006): 395–97.

————. "Multistate Outbreak of *Salmonella* Tennessee Infections Associated with Peanut Butter— United States, 2006–2007." *Morbidity and Mortality Weekly Report* 56, no. 21 (2007): 521–24.

————. "Norovirus Activity—United States, 2006–2007." *Morbidity and Mortality Weekly Reports* 56 (2007): 842–46, http://www.cdc.gov/mmwr/preview/mmwrhtml/mm5633a2.htm.

————. "Norovirus Outbreak among Evacuees from Hurricane Katrina—Houston, Texas, September, 2005." *Morbidity and Mortality Weekly Reports* 54, no. 40 (2005): 1016–18, http://www.cdc.gov/mmwr/preview/mmwrhtml/mm5440a3.htm.

————. "Norwalk-Like Viruses: Public Health Consequences and Outbreak Management." *Morbidity and Mortality Weekly Reports* 50, no. RR09 (2001), http://www.cdc.gov/mmwr/ preview/mmwrhtml/rr5009a1.htm.

————. "Outbreaks of Escherichia coli O157:H7 Infection and Cryptosporidiosis Associated with Drinking Unpasteurized Apple Cider—Connecticut and New York, October 1996." *Morbidity and Mortality Weekly Report* 46, no. 01 (1997): 4–8, http://www.cdc.gov/mmwr/ preview/mmwrhtml/00045558.htm.

————. "Preliminary FoodNet Data on the Incidence of Infection with Pathogens Transmitted Commonly through Food—10 States, 2006." *Morbidity and Mortality Weekly Report* 56, no. 14 (2007): 336–39.

————. "Public Health Dispatch: Outbreak of Listeriosis—Northeastern United States, 2002." *Morbidity and Mortality Weekly Report* 51, no. 42 (2002): 950–51, http://www.cdc.gov/ mmwr/preview/mmwrhtml/mm5142a3.htm.

————. "Rotavirus." http://www.cdc.gov/rotavirus/ (accessed January 8, 2008).

————. *Salmonella Surveillance: Annual Summary 2005.* http://www.cdc.gov/ncidod/dbmd/phlis data/salmonella.htm.

————. "Severe Methicillin-Resistant *Staphylococcus aureus* Community-Acquired Pneumonia Associated with Influenza—Louisiana and Georgia, December 2006—January 2007." *Morbidity and Mortality Weekly Reports* 56, no. 14 (2007): 325–29.

————. "Three Outbreaks of Salmonellosis Associated with Baby Poultry from Three Hatcheries—United States, 2006." *Morbidity and Mortality Weekly Report* 56, no. 12 (2007): 273–76.

————. *Traveler's Health Yellow Book.* http://wwwn.cdc.gov/travel/yellowBookCh4-Typhoid. aspx.

————. "Update: Listeriosis Outbreak Investigation." http://www.cdc.gov/od/oc/media/ pressrel/r021104.htm.

————. "Update—Outbreak of Cyclosporiasis United States and Canada, 1997." *Morbidity and Mortality Weekly Report* 46, no. 23 (1997): 521–23.

————. *Vessel Sanitation Operations Manual.* 2005. http://www.cdc.gov/nceh/vsp/operations manual/OPSManual2005.pdf.

————. "Youth Risk Behavioral Surveillance System." http://www.cdc.gov/HealthyYouth/yrbs/ index.htm.

Center for Food Safety and Nutrition. *CFSAN Budget Narrative.* 2008, http://www.fda.gov/oc/ oms/ofm/budget/2008/1-BudgetNarrativeCFSAN.pdf.

————. *Overview.* 2001. http://www.cfsan.fda.gov/~lrd/cfsan4.html.

————. *Produce Safety from Production to Consumption: 2004 Action Plan to Minimize Foodborne Illness Associated with Fresh Produce Consumption.* http://www.cfsan.fda.gov/~dms/prodpla2.html.

Center for Media and Democracy. "One Bad Apple? Facts and Myths Behind the 'Alar Scare.'" *PR Watch Newsletter,* second quarter 1997. http://www.prwatch.org/prwissues/1997Q2/alar.html.

Collinge, John, J. Whitfield, E. McKintosh, J. Beck, S. Mead, D. J. Thomas, and M. P. Alpers. "Kuru in the 21st Century—An Acquired Human Prion Disease with Very Long Incubation Periods." *The Lancet* 367 (2006): 2068–74.

Cools, I., M. Uyttendaele, J. Cerpentier, E. D'Haese, H. J. Nelis, and J. Debevere. "Persistence of *Campylobacter jejuni* on Surfaces in a Processing Environment and on Cutting Boards." *Letters in Applied Microbiology* 40 (2006): 418–23.

Crawford, Lester M. "BSE: A Veterinary History." In *The Mad Cow Crisis,* edited by Scott E. Ratzan, 14.

Cruise Line International Association. *The Cruise Industry, 2006 Economic Summary.* http://www.cruising.org/press/research/2006.CLIA.EconomicSummary.pdf.

Cuthbert, Jennifer A. "Hepatitis A: Old and New." *Clinical Microbiology Reviews* 14, no. 1 (2001): 38–58.

Davis, Margaret A., Thomas E. Besser, Kaye Eckmann, J. Kathryn MacDonald, Donna Green, Dale D. Hancock, Katherine N. K. Baker, Lorin D. Warnick, Yesim Soyer, Martin Wiedmann, and Douglas R. Call. "Multidrug-Resistant *Salmonella* Typhimurium, Pacific Northwest, United States." *Emerging Infectious Diseases* (2007), http://www.cdc.gov/eid/content/13/10/contents_v13n10.htm.

Dekeyser, P. M. Gossuin-Detrain, J. P. Butzler, and J. Sternon. "Acute Enteritis Due to Related *Vibrio*: First Positive Stool Cultures." *Journal of Infectious Diseases* 125 (1972): 390–92.

Dentinger, Catherine M., William A. Bower, Omana V. Nainan, Suzanne M. Cotter, Gert Myers, Letitia M. Dubusky, Suzanne Fowler, Ellen D. P. Salehi, and Beth P. Bell. "An Outbreak of Hepatitis A Associated with Green Onions." *The Journal of Infectious Diseases* 183 (2001): 1273–76.

De Reu, K., K. Grijspeerdt, W. Messens, M. Heyndrickx, M. Uyttendaele, J. Debevere, and L. Herman. "Eggshell Factors Influencing Eggshell Penetration and Whole Egg Contamination by Different Bacteria Including *Salmonella enteritidis.*" *International Journal of Food Microbiology* 112 (2006): 253–60.

Dhar, Rajat, Larry Stitt, and Angelika F. Hahn. "The Morbidity and Mortality of Patients with Guillain-Barré Syndrome Admitted to the Intensive Care Unit." *Journal of the Neurological Sciences* 264, no. 1/2 (2008): 121–28.

Doman, Claude E., and Richard J. Wolfe. *Suppressing the Diseases of Animals and Man: Theobald Smith, Microbiologist* (Boston: Harvard University Press, 2003).

Doyle, Ellin. *Foodborne Parasites: A Review of the Scientific Literature.* Madison, WI: UW: Food Research Institute, 2003, http://www.wisc.edu/fri/briefs/parasites.pdf.

Duckett, Serge, and Jan Stern. "Origins of the Creutzfeldt and Jakob Concept." *Journal of the History of the Neurosciences* 8, no. 1 (1999): 21–34.

Duffy, G., O. A. Lynch, and C. Cagney. "Tracking Emerging Zoonotic Pathogens From Farm to Fork." *Meat Science* 78 (2008): 34–42.

DuPont, Herbert L. "The Growing Threat of Foodborne Bacterial Enteropathogens of Animal Origin." *Clinical Infectious Diseases* 45 (2007): 1353–61.

Evans, M. R., C. D. Ribeiro, and R. L. Salmon. "Hazards of Healthy Living: Bottled Water and Salad Vegetables as Risk Factors for *Campylobacter* Infection." *Emerging Infectious Diseases* 9, no. 10 (2003): 1219–25.

Federal Register. "Scrapie in Sheep and Goats; Interstate Movement Restrictions and Indemnity Program; Final Rule." August 21, 2001.

Fenlon, David R. "Natural Environment." In *Listeria, Listeriosis, and Food Safety,* 2nd ed., edited by Elliot T. Ryser and Elmer H. Marth (New York: Marcel Dekker, 1999), 21–38.

Fiore, Anthony E. "Hepatitis A Transmitted by Food." *Clinical Infectious Diseases* 38 (2004): 705–15.

Fischer, Thea Kølsen, Nete Munk Nielsen, Jan Wohlfahrt, and Anders Pærregaard. "Incidence and Cost of Rotavirus Hospitalizations in Denmark." *Emerging Infectious Diseases* 13, no. 6 (2007), http://www.cdc.gov/eid/content/13/6/855.htm.

Food Safety Inspection Services. "Pathogen Reduction; Hazard Analysis and Critical Control Point (HACCP) Systems; Proposed Rule." *Federal Register* 60, no. 23 (February 3, 1995).

Fraser, Abigail, M. Paul, E. Goldberg, C. J. Acosta, and L. Leibovici. "Typhoid Fever Vaccines: Systematic Review and Meta-Analysis of Randomised Controlled Trials." *Vaccine* 25 (2007): 7848–57.

Friedman, Sharon, Kara Villamil, Robyn A. Suriano, and Brenda P. Egolf. "Alar and Apples: Newspapers, Risk and Media Responsibility." *Public Understanding of Science* 5 (1996): 1–20.

Fujikawa, H., H. Miyakawa, K. Iguchi, M. Nishizawa, K. Moro, K. Nagai, and M. Ishibashi. "Intestinal Cryptosporidiosis as an Initial Manifestation in a Previously Healthy Japanese Patient with AIDS." *Journal of Gastroenterology* 37 (2002): 840–43.

The Galileo Project. "Fracastoro, Girolamo." http://galileo.rice.edu/Catalog/NewFiles/fracstro.html.

Gandhi, Megha, and Karl R. Matthews. "Efficacy of Chlorine and Calcinated Calcium Treatment of Alfalfa Seeds and Sprouts to Eliminate Salmonella." *International Journal of Food Microbiology* 87, no. 3 (2003): 301–7.

Golan, Eloise, Fred Kuchler, Lorraine Mitchell, Cathy Greene, and Amber Jessup. *Economics of Food Labeling* (2001). http://www.ers.usda.gov/publications/aer793/.

Goldman, Emanuel. "Antibiotic Abuse in Animal Agriculture: Exacerbating Drug Resistance in Human Pathogens." *Human and Ecological Risk Assessment* 10 (2004): 121–34.

Government Accountability Office. *Mad Cow Disease: FDA's Management of the Feed Ban Has Improved, but Oversight Weaknesses Continue to Limit Program Effectiveness.* Washington, DC: GAO, 2005.

Gravani, Robert. "Incidence and Control of Listeria in Food-Processing Facilities." In *Listeria, Listeriosis, and Food Safety*, 2nd ed., edited by Elliot T. Ryser and Elmer H. Marth. New York: Marcel Dekker, 1999, 657–710.

Güerri, María Luisa, A. Aladueña, A. Echeíta, and R. Rotger. "Detection of Integrons and Antibiotic-Resistance Genes in *Salmonella enterica* serovar Typhimurium Isolates with Resistance to Ampicillin and Variable Susceptibility to Amoxicillin-Clavulanate." *International Journal of Antimicrobial Agents* 24 (2004): 327–33.

Haack, Jason P., Srdjan Jelacic, Thomas E. Besser, Edward Weinberger, Donald J. Kirk, Garry L. McKee, Shannon M. Harrison, Karl J. Musgrave, Gayle Miller, Thomas H. Price, and Phillip I. Tarr. "*Escherichia coli* O157 Exposure in Wyoming and Seattle: Serologic Evidence of Rural Risk." *Emerging Infectious Diseases* 9, no. 10 (2003): 1226–31.

Haaheim, L. R., J. R. Pattison, and Richard J. Whitley, eds. *A Practical Guide to Clinical Virology.* Chichester, NY: John Wiley & Sons, 2002. http://www.library.ohiou.edu:2326/Details.aspx (accessed January 9, 2008).

The Harris Poll. *CDC, FAA, NIH, FDA and FBI Get Highest Ratings of Eleven Federal Governing Agencies.* 2004, http://www.harrisinteractive.com/harris_poll/index.asp?PID=524.

Healy, Patrick. "Tormented by Viral Stowaway, Cruise Ship Staggers into Port." *New York Times,* September 3, 2005, B1.

Heyndrickx, Mark, F. Pasmans, R. Ducatelle, A. Decostere, and F. Haesebrouck. "Recent Changes in *Salmonella* Nomenclature: The Need for Clarification." *The Veterinary Journal* 170 (2005): 275–77.

Heywood P., J. Cutler, K. Burrows, C. Komorowski, B. Marshall, and H. L. Wang. "A Community Outbreak of Travel-Acquired Hepatitis A Transmitted by an Infected Food Handler." *Canada Communicable Disease Report* 1, no. 33 (2007): 16–23.

Hill Gaston, J. S., and M. S. Lillicrap. "Arthritis Associated with Enteric Infection." *Best Practice & Research. Clinical Rheumatology* 17 (2003): 219–39.

The History Guide. "Thucydides on the Athenian Plague of 430 B.C." http://www.historyguide. org/ancient/athenian_plague.html (accessed January 21, 2008).

Hoebe, Christian J. P.A., H. Vennema, A. M. de Roda Husman, and Y. T. van Duynhoven. "Norovirus Outbreak among Primary Schoolchildren Who Had Played in a Recreational Water Fountain." *Journal of Infectious Diseases* 189 (2004): 699–705.

Hof, H. "History and Epidemiology of Listeriosis." *FEMS Immunology and Medical Microbiology* 35 (2003): 199–202.

Holden, Costance. "Did FDR Have Guillain-Barré?" *Science* 302, no. 5647 (2003): 981.

Hu, Haijing, John J. Churey, and Randy W. Worobo. "Heat Treatments to Enhance the Safety of Mung Bean Seeds." *Journal of Food Protection* 67, no. 6 (2004): 1257–60.

Islam, Mahbub, J. Morgan, M. P. Doyle, and X. Jiang. "Survival of *Escherichia coli* O157:H7 in Soil and on Carrots and Onions Grown in Fields Treated with Contaminated Manure Composts or Irrigated Water." *Food Microbiology* 22 (2005): 63–70.

Janda, J. Michael, and Sharon L. Abbott. *The Enterobacteria* (Washington, DC: ASM Press, 2006).

Jay, James M. *Modern Food Microbiology.* 6th ed. (Gaithersburg, MD: Aspen, 2000).

Jay, Michele T., Michael Cooley, Diana Carychao, Gerald W. Wiscomb, Richard A. Sweitzer, Leta Crawford-Miksza, Jeff A. Farrar, David K. Lau, Janice O'Connell, Anne Millington, et al. "*Escherichia coli* O157:H7 in Feral Swine near Spinach Fields and Cattle, Central California Coast." *Emerging Infectious Disease Journal* (2007), http://www.cdc.gov/eid/content/13/12/1908.htm.

Karon, Amy E., John R. Archer, Mark J. Sotir, Timothy A. Monson, and James J. Kazmierczak. "Human Multi-Drug Resistant *Salmonella* Newport Infections, Wisconsin, 2003–2005." *Emerging Infectious Diseases* (2007), http://www.cdc.gov/eid/content/13/11/1777.htm.

Khan, Fahmi Yousef, A. A. Kamha, M. T. Abbas, F. Miyares, and S. S. Elshafie. "Guillain-Barré Syndrome Associated with *Salmonella paratyphi A*." *Clinical Neurology and Neurosurgery* 109 (2007): 452–54.

Kunin, Calvin M. "Urinary-Catheter-Associated Infections in the Elderly." *International Journal of Antimicrobial Agents* 28S (2006): S78–S81.

Larson, N. I., D. Neumark-Sztainer, P. J. Hannan, and M. Story. "Trends in Adolescent Fruit and Vegetable Consumption, 1999–2004: Project EAT." *American Journal of Preventive Medicine* 32 (2007): 147–50.

Lehr, Jay, and Sam Aldrich. "Alar: The Great Apple Scare." *Environment News*, March 1, 2007.

Leiss, William, and Douglas Powell. *Mad Cows and Mother's Milk: The Perils of Poor Risk Communication.* Quebec: McGill-Queen's University Press, 2004.

Levy, A. J. "A Gastro-enteritis Outbreak Probably Due to a Bovine Strain of *Vibrio*." *Journal of Infectious Diseases* 18 (1946): 243–58.

Lin, Jordan C. T., and Phil Kaufman. "Food Companies Offer View of Safe Handling Label for Meat and Poultry." *Food Review* (1995). http://findarticles.com/p/articles/mi_m3765/is_n3_v18/ai_18824581.

Loeffler, Friedrich, and P. Frosch. "Berichte der Kommission zur Erforschung der Maul-und Klauenseuche bei dem Institut fur Infektionskrankheiten." In *Milestones in Microbiology: 1556 to 1940*, translated and edited by Thomas D. Brock. ASM Press, 1998: 149.

Lorimer, George Hormis. "Servant of Mankind." *Saturday Evening Post* 207, no. 37 (1935): 26.

Luber, P., and E. Bartelt. "Enumeration of *Campylobacter* spp. on the Surface and within Chicken Breast Fillets." *Journal of Applied Microbiology* 102 (2007): 313–18.

Luber, P., S. Brynestad, D. Topsch, K. Scherer, and E. Bartelt. "Quantification of *Campylobacter* Species Cross-contamination During Handling of Contaminated Fresh Chicken Parts in Kitchens." *Applied and Environmental Microbiology* 72, no. 91 (2006): 66–70.

Lyman, Howard. *Oprah Winfrey Show* transcript. April 15, 1996. http://www.vegsource.com/lyman/oprah_transcript.htm.

Manuelidis, Laura, Zhoa-Xue Yu, Nuria Barquero, and Brian Mullins. "Cells Infected with Scrapie and Creutzfeldt-Jakob Disease Agents Produce Intracellular 25-nm Virus-Like Particles." *Proceedings of the National Academy of Sciences* 104, no. 6 (2007): 1965–70.

Marks, P. J., I. B. Vipond, D. Carlisle, D. Deakin, R. E. Fey, and E. O. Caul. "Evidence for Airborne Transmission of Norwalk-Like Virus in a Hotel Restaurant." *Epidemiology and Infection* 124 (2000): 481–87.

McLauchlin, J., R. T. Mitchell, W. J. Smerdon, and K. Jewell. "*Listeria monocytogenes* and Listeriosis: A Review of Hazard Characterization for Use in Microbiological Risk Assessment of Foods." *International Journal of Food Microbiology* 94 (2004): 15–33.

McLaughlin, Joseph B., A. DePaola, C. A. Bopp, K. A. Martinek, N. P. Napolilli, C. G. Allison, S. L. Murray, E. C. Thompson, M. M. Bird, and J. P. Middaugh. "Outbreak of *Vibrio parahaemolyticus* Gastroenteritis Associated with Alaskan Oysters." *The New England Journal of Medicine* 353, no. 14 (2005): 1463–70.

Medline Plus Medical Encyclopedia. "Typhoid Fever." http://www.nlm.nih.gov/medlineplus/ency/article/001332.htm (accessed January 21, 2008).

Meisle, J. L., D. R. Perera, C. Meligro, and C. E. Rubin. "Overwhelming Watery Diarrhea Associated with *Cryptosporidium* in and Immunocompromised Patient." *Gastroenterology* 70 (1976): 1156–60.

Murray, E.G.D., R. A. Webb, and H.B.R. Swann. "A Disease of Rabbits Characterized by a Hitherto Undescribed Bacillus *Bacterium monocytogenes* (n. sp.)." *Journal of Pathology and Bacteriology* 29 (1926): 407–39.

Nanji, Shabin S. "Cruise Ships, Oysters, and Edible Vaccines: Revisiting the Non-cultivable Norwalk-Like Virus Responsible for Outbreaks of Gastroenteritis." *Clinical Microbiology Newsletter* 26 (2004): 1–4.

National Advisory Committee on Microbiological Criteria for Food. *Microbiological Safety Evaluation and Recommendations on Sprouted Seeds.* http://www.cfsan.fda.gov/~mow/sprouts2.html.

National Archives. *Records of the Bureau of Animal Industry.* http://www.archives.gov/research/guide-fed-records/groups/017.html#17.

Natural Resources Defense Council. "Intolerable Risk: Pesticides in Our Children's Food." February 27, 1989. http://tobaccodocuments.org/pm/2025546150-6160.html (accessed January 17, 2008).

Neira, Maria. "Cholera: A Challenge for the 21st Century." *World Health* 50 (1997): 9.

Nime, F. A., J. D. Burek, D. L. Page, M. A. Holscher, and J. H. Yardley. "Acute Enterocolitis in a Human Being Infected with the Protozoan *Cryptosporidium*." *Gastroenterology* 70 (1976): 592–98.

Papagrigorakis, Manolis J., Christos Yapijakis, Philippos N. Synodinos, and Effie Baziotopoulou-Valavani. "DNA Examination of Ancient Dental Pulp Incriminates Typhoid Fever as Probable Cause of the Plague of Athens." *International Journal of Infectious Diseases* 10 (2006): 206–14.

Papagrigorakis, Manolis J., Philippos N. Synodinos, and Christos Yapijakis. "Ancient Typhoid Epidemic Reveals Possible Ancestral Strain of *Salmonella enterica* serovar Typhi." *Infection, Genetics and Evolution* 7 (2007): 126–27.

Parachin, Victor M. "Typhoid Mary: 'The Most Dangerous Woman in America'." *American History* 40 (2006): 24–26.

Park, Y., A. F. Subar, V. Kipnis, F. E. Thompson, T. Mouw, A. Hollenbeck, M. F. Leitzmann, and A. Schatzkin. "Fruit and Vegetable Intakes and Risk of Colorectal Cancer in the NIH–AARP Diet and Health Study." *American Journal of Epidemiology* 166 (2007): 170–80.

Paul, Mathilde, David Abrial, Nathalie Jarrige, Stéphane Rican, Myriam Garrido, Didier Calavas, and Christian Ducrot. "Bovine Spongiform Encephalopathy and Spatial Analysis of the Feed Industry." *Emerging Infectious Diseases* 13, no. 6 (2007), http://www.cdc.gov/eid/content/13/6/contents_v13n06.htm.

Pedersen, Joel A., Katherine D. McMahon, and Craig H. Benson. "Prions: Novel Pathogens of Environmental Concern?" *Journal of Environmental Engineering* (2006): 967–69.

Philips, Matthew. "They're Seeing Red over Greens." *Newsweek* 148 (October 2, 2006): 14.

Pirie, James Hunter Harvey. "*Listeria*: Change of Name for a Genus of Bacteria." *Nature* 145, no. 3668: 264.

Prusiner, Stanley B. "Detecting Mad Cow Disease." *Scientific American* 291, no. 1 (2004): 88.

Punda-Polić, Volga, K. S. Kraljević, and N. Bradarić. "War-Associated Cases of Typhoid Fever Imported to Split-Dalmatia County (Croatia). *Military Medicine* 172, no. 10 (2007): 1096–98.

Punzi, L., M. Pianon, A. Pozzuoli, F. Oliviero, G. P. Salvati, and P. F. Gambari. "Psoriatic Arthritis Exacerbated by *Salmonella* Infection." *Clinical Rheumatology* 19 (2000): 167–68.

Ratzan, Scott C. *The Mad Cow Crisis.* New York: New York University Press, 1998, ix.

Reynolds, Dennis, and William M. Balinbin. "Mad Cow Disease: An Empirical Investigation of Restaurant Strategies and Consumer Response." *Journal of Hospitality & Tourism Research* 27, no. 3 (2003): 358–68.

Rocourt, Jocelyn. "The Genus *Listeria* and *Listeria monocytogenes*: Phylogenetic Position, Taxonomy, and Identification." In *Listeria, Listeriosis, and Food Safety*, 2nd ed., edited by Elliot T. Ryser and Elmer H. Marth. New York: Marcel Dekker, 1999, 1–20.

Rott, Rudolf, and Stuart Siddell. "One Hundred Years of Animal Virology." *Journal of General Virology* 79 (1998): 2871–74.

Roumagnac, Philippe, François-Xavier Weill, Christiane Dolecek, Stephen Baker, Sylvain Brisse, Nguyen Tran Chinh, Thi Anh Hong Le, Camilo J. Acosta, Jeremy Farrar, and Gordon Dougan. "Evolutionary History of *Salmonella* Typhi." *Science* 314: 1301–4.

Ryser, Elliot T. "Foodborne Listeriosis." In *Listeria, Listeriosis, and Food Safety*, 2nd ed., edited by Elliot T. Ryser and Elmer H. Marth. New York: Marcel Dekker, 1999, 299–358.

Sanchez-Juan, Pascual, N. Cousens, Robert G. Will, and Cornelia M. van Duijn. "Source of Variant Creutzfeldt-Jakob Disease outside the United Kingdom." *Emerging Infectious Diseases* 13, no. 8 (2007): 1166–68.

Saroj, Sunil D., R. Shashidhar, M. Pandey, V. Dhokane, S. Hajare, A. Sharma, and J. R. Bandekar. "Effectiveness of Radiation Processing in Elimination of *Salmonella typhimurium* and *Listeria monocytogenes* from Sprouts." *Journal of Food Protection* 69, no. 8 (2006): 1858–64.

Saxbe, W. B., Jr. "*Listeria monocytogenes* and Queen Anne." *Pediatrics* 49, no. 1 (1972): 97–101.

Schink, Bernhard. "Hans Günter Schlegel 80 Years Old." *Archives of Microbiology* 182 (2004): 103–4.

Schlegel, Hans G. "Continuing Opportunities for General Microbiology." *Archives of Microbiology* 182 (2004): 107.

Seeliger, Heinz P. R. *Listeriosis.* New York: Hafner, 1961.

Senate Committee on Science, Commerce, and Transportation. *Mad Cow Disease: Are Our Precautions Adequate?* 107th Cong., 1st sess. 2001, http://bulk.resource.org/gpo.gov/hearings/107s/88461.pdf.

Setbon, Michel, Jocelyn Raude, Claude Fischler, and Antoine Flahault. "Risk Perception of the 'Mad Cow Disease' in France: Determinant and Consequences." *Risk Analysis* 25, no. 4 (2005): 813–26.

Seto, Edmund Y. W., Jeffrey A. Soller, and John M. Colford, Jr. "Strategies to Reduce Person-to-Person Transmission during Widespread *Escherichia coli* O157:H7 Outbreak." *Emerging Infectious Diseases* 13, no. 6 (2007), http://www.cdc.gov/eid/content/13/6/860.htm.

Shapiro, Beth, Andrew Rambaut, and M. Thomas P. Gilbert. "No Proof that Typhoid Causes the Plague of Athens (A Reply to Papagrigorakis et al.)." *International Journal of Infectious Diseases* 10 (2006): 334–340.

Shulman, Stanford T., Herbert C. Friedmann, and Ronald H. Sims. "Theodor Escherich: The First Pediatric Infectious Disease Physician?" *Clinical Infectious Diseases* 45, no. 8 (2007): 1025–29.

Slaughter, Adele. "Meryl Streep Takes a Lead in Environmental Health." *USA Today*, October 18, 2002, http://www.usatoday.com/news/health/spotlighthealth/2002-10-18-streep-healthy-kids_x.htm.

Smith, H. V., S. M. Cacciò, N. Cook, R. A. Nichols, and A. Tait. "Cryptosporidium and Giardia as Foodborne Zoonoses." *Veterinary Parasitology* 149 (2007): 29–40.

Steinberg, E. B., R. Bishop, P. Haber, A. F. Dempsey, R. M. Hoekstra, J. M. Nelson, M. Ackers, A. Calugar, E. D. Mintz. "Typhoid Fever in Travelers: Who Should Be Targeted for Prevention?" *Clinical Infectious Diseases* 39 (2004):186–91.

Su, Yi-Cheng, and Chengchu Liu. "*Vibrio parahaemolyticus:* A Concern for Seafood Safety." *Food Microbiology* 24 (2007): 549–58.

Swaminathan, Bala, and Peter Gerner-Smidt. "The Epidemiology of Human Listeriosis." *Microbes and Infection* 9 (2007): 1236–43.

Tindall, B. J., P. A. Grimont, G. M. Garrity, and J. P. Euzéby. "Nomenclature and Taxonomy of the Genus *Salmonella.*" *International Journal of Systemic and Evolutionary Microbiology* 55 (2005): 521–24.

Tyzzer, Edward. "A Sporozoan Found in the Peptic Glands of the Common Mouse." *Proceedings of the Society for Experimental Biology and Medicine* 5 (1907): 12–13.

Tzipori, Sauonorine, and H. Ward. "Cryptosporidiosis: Biology, Pathogenesis and Disease." *Microbes and Infection* 4 (2002): 1047–58.

U.S. Department of Agriculture. "Enforcement, Investigations, and Analysis Officer (EIAO) Assessment of Compliance with the Listeria Monocytogenes (Lm) Regulation and Introduction of Phase 2 of the Lm Risk-Based Verification Testing Program." 2006. http://www.fsis.usda.gov/OPPDE/rdad/FSISDirectives/10240.5.pdf.

———. *FY 2008 Budget Summary and Annual Performance Plan.* http://www.obpa.usda.gov/budsum/fy08budsum.pdf (accessed January 15, 2008).

———. *NAHMS Scrapie: Ovine Slaughter Surveillance (SOSS) Study 2001–2003.* http://www.aphis.usda.gov/animal_health/animal_diseases/scrapie/downloads/sossphase2.pdf.

———. Safe Handling Label Text. http://www.fsis.usda.gov/News/Safe_Handling_Label_Text/index.asp.

U.S. Department of Health and Human Services. *Dietary Guidelines for Americans.* http://www.health.gov/dietaryguidelines/.

U.S. Department of Health Education and Welfare. *Healthy People: The Surgeon General's Report on Health Promotion and Disease Prevention.* Washington, DC: U.S. Government Printing Office, 1979. http://profiles.nlm.nih.gov/NN/B/B/G/K/_/nnbbgk.pdf.

U.S. Environmental Protection Agency. "Daminozide (Alar) Pesticide Canceled for Food Uses." Press release. November 7, 1989. http://www.epa.gov/history/topics/food/02.htm.

U.S. Food and Drug Administration. *Bad Bug Book.* http://www.cfsan.fda.gov/~mow/intro.html.

———. FDA Press Conference on Chili Products (Botulism) Recall. July 24, 2007. http://www.fda.gov/bbs/transcripts/transcript072407.pdf.

———. "FDA Update on Recent Hepatitis A Outbreaks Associated with Green Onions from Mexico." December 9, 2003. http://www.fda.gov/bbs/topics/NEWS/2003/NEW00993.html (accessed January 10, 2008).

———. *Quantitative Assessment of Relative Risk to Public Health from Foodborne Listeria monocytogenes among Selected Categories of Ready-to-eat Foods.* 2003. http://www.cfsan.fda.gov/~dms/lmr2-toc.html.

———. *Quantitative Risk Assessment on the Public Health Impact of Vibrio parahaemolyticus in Raw Oysters.* 2005. http://www.cfsan.fda.gov/%7Edms/vpra-toc.html (accessed January 10, 2008).

U.S. House of Representatives, Subcommittee on Science and Technology. *FDA Science and Mission at Risk.* December 3, 2007. http://www.fda.gov/ohrms/dockets/ac/07/briefing/2007-4329b_02_00_index.html.

Van, Thi Thu Hao, George Moutafis, Taghrid Istivan, Linh Thuoc Tran, and Peter J. Coloe. "Detection of *Salmonella* spp. in Retail Raw Food Samples from Vietnam and Characterization of Their Antibiotic Resistance." *Applied and Environmental Microbiology* 73 (2007): 6885–90.

The Wall Street Journal. "How a PR Firm Executed the Alar Scare." October 3, 1989, Section 1, 22.

Wasley, Annemarie, Jeremy T. Miller, and Lyn Finelli. "Surveillance for Acute Viral Hepatitis—United States, 2005." *Morbidity and Mortality Weekly Report* 56, no. SS03 (2007): 1–24.

Weeks, Jennifer. "Factory Farms: Are They the Best Way to Feed the Nation?" *CQ Researcher* 17, no. 2 (2007), http://library.cqpress.com/cqresearcher/cqresrre2007011200.

Weiss, Linda, Elizabeth Thurbon, and John Mathews. "Free Trade in Mad Cows: How to Kill a Beef Industry." *Australian Journal of International Affairs* 60, no. 1 (2006): 376–99.

Weller, Thomas H. *Ernest Edward Tyzzer: A Biographical Memoir.* Washington, DC: National Academy of Sciences, 1978.

Wheeler, C., Tara M. Vogt, Gregory L. Armstrong, Gilberto Vaughan, Andre Weltman, Omana V. Nainan, Virginia Dato, Guoliang Xia, Kirsten Waller, Joseph Amon, et al. "An Outbreak of Hepatitis A Associated with Green Onions." *New England Journal of Medicine* 353 (2005): 890–97.

White House, Office of the Press Secretary. "President Clinton Announces Aggressive Food Safety Strategy to Combat Listeria in Hot Dogs and Other Ready-To-Eat Foods." May 6, 2000. http://www.foodsafety.gov/~dms/fs-wh20.html.

Whonamedit.com. "Daniel Salmon." http://www.whonamedit.com/doctor.cfm/408.html (accessed January 21, 2008).

Will, R. G., and J. W. Ironside. "A New Variant of Creutzfeldt-Jakob in the UK." *The Lancet* 347 (1996): 921–25.

World Health Organization. "Cholera, 2005." *Weekly Epidemiological Record* 31 (2006): 297–308.

———. *Epidemic and Pandemic Alert and Response: Hepatitis A.* http://www.who.int/csr/disease/hepatitis/whocdscsredc2007/en/index4.html#worldwide (accessed January 10, 2008).

———. *Global Polio Eradication Initiative: The History.* http://www.polioeradication.org/history.asp#1789 (accessed January 10, 2008).

———. *Global Salm Surv.* http://www.who.int/salmsurv/en/ (accessed January 9, 2008).

———. *WHO Global Salm-Surv Strategic Plan 2006–2010* (Geneva, Switzerland: WHO, 2006), http://www.who.int/salmsurv/general/documents/GSS_STRATEGICPLAN2006_10.pdf.

Yan, S. Steve, et al. "*Campylobacter* Infection and Guillain-Barré Syndrome: Public Health Concerns from a Microbial Food Safety Perspective." *Clinical and Applied Immunology Reviews* 5 (2005): 285–305.

Yoder, Jonathan S., and Michael J. Beach. "Cryptosporidiosis Surveillance—United States, 2003–2005." *Morbidity and Mortality Weekly Report* 56, no. SS05 (2007): 1–10, http://www.cdc.gov/mmwr/preview/mmwrhtml/ss5607a1.htm.

Zimmerman, A. M., A. DePaola, J. C. Bowers, J. A. Krantz, J. L. Nordstrom, C. N. Johnson, and D. J. Grimes. "Variability of Total and Pathogenic *Vibrio parahaemolyticus* Densities in Northern Gulf of Mexico Water and Oysters." *Applied and Environmental Microbiology* 73, no. 23 (2007): 7589–96.

FURTHER READING

Doman, Claude E., and Richard J. Wolfe. *Suppressing the Diseases of Animals and Man: Theobald Smith, Microbiologist*. Boston: Harvard University Press, 2003.

Garrity, George M., ed. *Bergey's Manual of Systematic Bacteriology*, 2nd ed. New York: Springer, 2001.

Heritage, J., E.G.V. Evans, and R. A. Killington. *Introductory Microbiology*. London: Cambridge University Press, 1996.

Janda, J. Michael. *The Enterobacteria*. 2nd ed. Washington, DC: ASM, 2006.

Jay, James M. *Modern Food Microbiology*. 6th ed. Gaithersburg, MD: Aspen, 2000.

Motarjem, Yasmine, and Martin Adams, eds. *Emerging Foodborne Pathogens*. Cambridge, UK: Woodhead Publishing, 2006.

Ratzan, Scott G., ed. *The Mad Cow Crisis: Health and the Public Good*. New York: New York University Press, 1998.

Ryser, Elliot T. and Elmer H. Marth, ed. *Listeria, Listeriosis, and Food Safety*. 2nd ed. New York: Marcel Dekker, 1999.

U.S. Food and Drug Administration. *Bad Bug Book*. http://www.cfsan.fda.gov/~mow/intro.html.

Vinten-Johansen, Peter, Howard Brody, Nigel Paneth, Stephen Rackman, and Michael Rip. *Cholera, Chloroform and the Science of Medicine: A Life of John Snow*. New York: Oxford University Press, 2003.

Wagner, Edward K., and Martinez J. Hewlett. *Basic Virology*. Malden, MA: Blackwell, 1999.

Walters, Mark Jerome. *Six Modern Plagues and How We are Causing Them*. Washington, DC: Island Press, 2003.

Index

About the Author

MICHELE MORRONE is Associate Professor of Environmental Health Science and the Director of Environmental Studies at Ohio University in Athens, Ohio. She is a registered sanitarian and a credentialed food safety professional. She is the past Chief of the Ohio Environmental Protection Agency's Office of Environmental Education and has served on the boards of numerous environmental organizations. She has authored or co-authored more than 45 publications on issues related to educating the public about environmental health risks, including *Sound Science, Junk Policy: Environmental Health Science and the Decision-Making Process* (Greenwood, 2002).